THE DARK LETTER

THE DORÉ LECTURES

BOOKS BY THOMAS TROWARD

Bible Mystery and Bible Meaning
The Creative Process in the Individual
The Doré Lectures
The Edinburgh Lectures
The Law and the Word
The Hidden Power

THE
DORÉ LECTURES

Being Sunday Addresses at the Doré
Gallery, London, Given in Connection
with the Higher Thought Centre, 10,
Cheniston Gardens, Kensington.

by Thomas Troward

Fides et Amor Veritas et Robur

DODD, MEAD & COMPANY
NEW YORK

CONTENTS.

FOREWORD.

THE addresses contained in this volume were delivered by me at the Doré Gallery, Bond Street, London, on the Sundays of the first three months of the present year, and are now published at the kind request of many of my hearers, hence their title of "The Doré Lectures." A number of separate discourses on a variety of subjects necessarily labours under the disadvantage of want of continuity, and also under that of a liability to the frequent repetition of similar ideas and expressions, and the reader will, I trust, pardon these defects as inherent in the circumstances of the work. At the same time it will be found that, although not specially so designed, there is a certain progressive development of thought through the dozen lectures which compose this volume, the reason for which is that they all aim at expressing the same fundamental idea, namely that, though the laws of the universe can never be broken, they can be made to work under special conditions which will produce results that could not be produced under the conditions spontaneously provided by nature. This is a simple scientific principle and it shows us the place which is occupied by the personal factor, that, namely, of an intelligence which sees beyond the present limited manifestation of the Law into its real essence, and which thus constitutes the instrumentality by which the infinite possibilities of the Law can be evoked into forms of power, usefulness, and beauty.

The more perfect, therefore, the working of the personal factor, the greater will be the results developed from the Universal Law; and hence our lines of study should be two-fold—on the one hand the theoretical study of the action of Universal Law, and on the other the practical fitting of ourselves to make use of it; and if the present volume should assist any reader in this two-fold quest, it will have answered its purpose.

The different subjects have necessarily been treated very briefly, and the addresses can only be considered as suggestions for lines of thought which the reader will be able to work out for himself, and he must therefore not expect that careful elaboration of detail which I would gladly have bestowed had I been writing on one of these subjects exclusively. This little book must be taken only for what it is, the record of somewhat fragmentary talks with a very indulgent audience, to whom I gratefully dedicate the volume.

T.T.

JUNE 5, 1909.

THE DORÉ LECTURES

ENTERING INTO THE SPIRIT OF IT.

WE all know the meaning of this phrase in our everyday life. The Spirit is that which gives life and movement to anything, in fact it is that which causes it to exist at all. The thought of the author, the impression of the painter, the feeling of the musician, is that without which their works could never have come into being, and so it is only as we enter into the *idea* which gives rise to the work, that we can derive all the enjoyment and benefit from it which it is able to bestow. If we cannot enter into the Spirit of it, the book, the picture, the music, are meaningless to us: to appreciate them we must share the mental attitude of their creator. This is a universal principle; if we do not enter into the Spirit of a thing, it is dead so far as we are concerned; but if we do enter into it we reproduce in ourselves the same quality of life which called that thing into existence.

Now if this is a general principle, why can we not carry it to a higher range of things? Why not to the highest point of all? May we not enter into the originating Spirit of Life itself, and so reproduce it in ourselves as a perennial spring of livingness? This, surely, is a question worthy of our careful consideration.

The spirit of a thing is that which is the source of its inherent movement, and therefore the question before us is, what is the nature of the primal moving power, which is at the back of the endless array of life which we see around us, our own life included? Science gives us ample ground for saying that it is not material, for science has now, at least theoretically, reduced all material things to a primary ether, universally distributed, whose innumerable particles are in absolute equilibrium; whence it follows on mathematical grounds alone that the initial movement which began to concentrate the world and all material substances out of the particles of the dispersed ether, could not have originated in the particles themselves. Thus by a necessary deduction from the conclusions of physical science, we are compelled to realize the presence of some immaterial power capable of separating off certain specific areas for the display of cosmic activity, and then building up a material universe with all its inhabitants by an orderly sequence of evolution, in which each stage lays the foundation for the development of the stage, which is to follow—in a word we find ourselves brought face to face with a power which exhibits on a stupendous scale, the faculties of selection and adaptation of means to ends, and thus distributes energy and life in accordance with a recognizable scheme of cosmic progression. It is therefore not only Life, but also Intelligence, and Life guided by Intelligence becomes Volition. It is this primary originating power which we mean when we speak of " The Spirit," and it is into this Spirit of the whole universe that we must enter if we would reproduce it as a spring of Original Life in ourselves.

Now in the case of the productions of artistic genius we know that we must enter into the movement of the creative mind of the artist, before we can realize the principle which gives rise to his work. We must learn to partake of the feeling, to find expression for which is the motive of his creative activity. May we not apply the same principle to the Greater Creative Mind with which we are seeking to deal? There is something in the work of the artist which is akin to that of original creation. His work, literary, musical, or graphic is original creation on a miniature scale, and in this it differs from that of the engineer, which is constructive, or that of the scientist which is analytical; for the artist in a sense creates something out of nothing, and therefore starts from the stand-point of simple feeling, and not from that of a pre-existing necessity. This, by the hypothesis of the case, is true also of the Parent Mind, for at the stage where the initial movement of creation takes place, there are no existing conditions to compel action in one direction more than another. Consequently the direction taken by the creative impulse is not dictated by outward circumstances, and the primary movement must therefore be entirely due to the action of the Original Mind upon itself; it is the reaching out of this Mind for realization of all that it feels itself to be.

The creative process thus in the first instance is purely a matter of feeling—exactly what we speak of as "motif" in a work of art.

Now it is this original feeling that we need to enter into, because it is the *fons et origo* of the whole chain of causation which subsequently follows. What then can this original feeling of the Spirit be? Since the Spirit is Life-in-itself, its feeling can only be for the fuller expression of Life— any other sort of feeling would be self-destructive and is therefore inconceivable. Then the full expression of Life implies Happiness, and Happiness implies Harmony, and Harmony implies Order, and Order implies Proportion, and Proportion implies Beauty; so that in recognizing the inherent tendency of the Spirit towards the production of Life, we can recognise a similar inherent tendency to the production of these other qualities also; and since the desire to bestow the greater fulness of joyous life can only be described as Love, we can sum up the whole of the feeling which is the original moving impulse in the Spirit as Love and Beauty—the Spirit finding expression through forms of beauty in centres of life, in harmonious reciprocal relation to itself. This is a generalized statement of the broad principle by which Spirit expands from the innermost to the outermost, in accordance with a Law of tendency inherent in itself.

It sees itself, as it were, reflected in various centres of life and energy, each with its appropriate form; but in the first instance these reflections can have no existence except within the originating Mind. They have their first beginning as mental images, so that in addition to the powers of Intelligence and Selection, we must also realise that of Imagination as belonging to the Divine Mind; and we must picture these powers as working from the initial motive of Love and Beauty.

Now this is the Spirit that we need to enter into, and the method of doing so is a perfectly logical one. It is the same method by which all scientific advance is made. It consists in first observing how a certain law works under the conditions spontaneously provided by nature, next in carefully considering what principle this spontaneous working indicates, and lastly deducing from this how the same principle would act under specially selected conditions, not spontaneously provided by nature.

The progress of shipbuilding affords a good example of what I mean. Formerly wood was employed instead of iron, because wood floats in water and iron sinks; yet now the navies of the world are built of iron; careful thought showed the law of floatation to be that anything could float which, bulk for bulk, is lighter than the mass of liquid displaced by it; and so we now make iron float by the very same law by which it sinks, because by the introduction of the *personal* factor, we provide conditions which do not occur spontaneously—according to the esoteric maxim that " Nature unaided fails." Now we want to apply the same process of specializing a generic Law to the first of all Laws, that of the generic life-giving tendency of Spirit itself. Without the element of *individual personality* the Spirit can only work cosmically by a *generic* Law; but this law admits of far higher specialization, and this specialization can only be attained through the introduction of the personal factor. But to introduce this factor the individual must be fully aware of the *principle* which underlies the spontaneous or cosmic action of the law. Where, then, will he find this principle of Life? Certainly not by contemplating Death. In order to get a principle to work in the way we require it to, we must observe its action when it is working spontaneously in this particular direction. We must ask why it goes in the right direction as far as it does—and having learnt this we shall then be able to make it go further. The law of floatation was not discovered by contemplating the sinking of things, but by contemplating the floating of things which floated naturally, and then intelligently asking why they did so.

The knowledge of a principle is to be gained by the study of its affirmative action; when we understand *that* we are in a position to correct the negative conditions which tend to prevent that action.

Now Death is the absence of Life, and disease is the absence of health, so to enter into the Spirit of Life we require to contemplate it, where it is to be found, and not where it is not—we are met with the old question, " Why seek ye the living among the dead? " This is why we start our studies by considering the cosmic creation, for it is there that we find the Life Spirit working through untold ages, not merely as deathless energy, but with a perpetual advance into higher degrees of Life. If we could only so enter into the Spirit as to make it personally *in ourselves* what it evidently is in *itself*, the *magnum opus* would be accomplished. This means realizing our life as drawn direct from the Originating Spirit; and if we now understand that the Thought or Imagination of the Spirit is the great reality of Being, and that all material facts are only correspondences, then it logically follows that what we have to do is to maintain our individual place in the Thought of the Parent Mind.

We have seen that the action of the Originating Mind must needs be *generic*, that is according to types which include multitudes of individuals. This type is the reflection of the Creative Mind at the level of that particular *genius;* and at the human level it is Man, not as associated with particular circumstances, but as existing in the absolute ideal.

In proportion then as we learn to dissociate our conception of ourselves from particular circumstances, and to rest upon our *absolute* nature, as reflections of the Divine ideal, we, in our turn, reflect back into the Divine Imagination its original conception of itself as expressed in generic or typical Man, and so by a natural law of cause and effect, the individual who realizes this mental attitude enters permanently into the Spirit of Life, and it becomes a perennial fountain of Life springing up spontaneously within him.

He then finds himself to be as the Bible says, "the image and likeness of God." He has reached the level at which he affords a new starting point for the creative process, and the Spirit, finding a personal centre in him, begins its work *de novo,* having thus solved the great problem of how to enable the Universal to act directly upon the plane of the Particular.

It is in this sense, as affording the requisite centre for a new departure of the creative Spirit, that man is said to be a " microcosm," or universe in miniature; and this is also what is meant by the esoteric doctrine of the Octave, of which I may be able to speak more fully on some other occasion.

If the principles here stated are carefully considered, they will be found to throw light on much that would otherwise be obscure, and they will also afford the key to the succeeding essays.

The reader is therefore asked to think them out carefully for himself, and to note their connection with the subject of the next article.

INDIVIDUALITY.

INDIVIDUALITY is the necessary complement of the Universal Spirit, which was the subject of our consideration last Sunday. The whole problem of life consists in finding the true relation of the individual to the Universal Originating Spirit; and the first step towards ascertaining this is to realize what the Universal Spirit must be in itself. We have already done this to some extent, and the conclusions we have arrived at are:—

That the essence of the Spirit is Life, Love, and Beauty.

That its Motive, or primary moving impulse, is to express the Life, Love and Beauty which it feels itself to be.

That the Universal cannot act on the plane of the Particular except by becoming the particular, that is by expression through the individual.

If these three axioms are clearly grasped, we have got a solid foundation from which to start our consideration of the subject for to-day.

The first question that naturally presents itself is,

If these things be so, why does not every individual express the life, love, and beauty of the Universal Spirit? The answer to this question is to be found in the Law of Consciousness. We cannot be conscious of anything except by realizing a certain relation between it and ourselves. It must affect us in some way, otherwise we are not conscious of its existence; and according to the way in which it affects us we recognize ourselves as standing related to it. It is this self-recognition on our own part carried out to the sum total of all our relations, whether spiritual, intellectual, or physical, that constitutes our realization of life. On this principle, then, for the *realization* of its own Livingness, the production of centres of life, through its relation to which this conscious realization can be attained, becomes a necessity for the Originating Mind. Then it follows that this realization can only be complete where the individual has perfect liberty to withhold it; for otherwise no true realization could have taken place. For instance, let us consider the working of Love. Love must be spontaneous, or it has no existence at all. We cannot imagine such a thing as mechanically induced love. But anything which is formed so as to automatically produce an effect without any volition of its own, is nothing but a piece of mechanism. Hence if the Originating Mind is to realize the reality of Love, it can only be by relation to some being which has the power to withhold love. The same applies to the realization of all the other modes of livingness; so that it is only in proportion, as the individual life is an independent centre of action, with the option of acting either positively or negatively, that any real life has been produced at all. The further the created thing is from being a merely mechanical arrangement, the higher is the grade of creation. The solar system is a perfect work of mechanical creation, but to constitute centres which can reciprocate the highest nature of the Divine Mind, requires not a mechanism, however perfect, but a mental centre which is, in itself, an independent source of action. Hence by the requirements of the case man should be capable of placing himself either in a positive or a negative relation to the Parent Mind, from which he originates; otherwise he would be nothing more than a clockwork figure.

In this necessity of the case, then, we find the reason why the life, love, and beauty of the Spirit are not visibly reproduced in every human being. They *are* reproduced in the world of nature, so far as a mechanical and automatic action can represent them, but their perfect reproduction can only take place on the basis of a liberty akin to that of the Originating Spirit itself, which therefore implies the liberty of negation as well as of affirmation.

Why, then, does the individual make a negative choice? Because he does not understand the law of his own individuality, and believes it to be a law of limitation, instead of a Law of Liberty. He does not expect to find the starting point of the Creative Process reproduced within himself, and so he looks to the mechanical side of things for the basis of his reasoning about life. Consequently his reasoning lands him in the conclusion that life is limited, because he has assumed limitation in his premises, and so logically cannot escape from it in his conclusion. Then he thinks that this is the law and so ridicules the idea of transcending it. He points to the sequence of cause and effect, by which death, disease, and disaster, hold their sway over the individual, and says that sequence is law. And he is perfectly right so far as he goes—it is *a* law; but not *the* Law. When we have only reached this stage of comprehension, we have yet to learn that a higher law can include a lower one so completely as entirely to swallow it up.

The fallacy involved in this negative argument, is the assumption that the law of limitation is essential in all grades of being. It is the fallacy of the old shipbuilders as to the impossibility of building iron ships. What is required is to get at the *principle* which is at the back of the Law in its affirmative working, and specialize it under higher conditions than are spontaneously presented by nature, and this can only be done by the introduction of the personal element, that is to say an individual intelligence capable of comprehending the principle. The question, then, is, what is the principle by which we came into being? and this is only a personal application of the general question, How did anything come into being? Now, as I pointed out in the preceding article, the ultimate deduction from physical science is that the originating movement takes place in the Universal Mind, and is analogous to that of our own imagination; and as we have just seen, the perfect ideal can only be that of a being capable of reciprocating *all* the qualities of the Originating Mind. Consequently man, in his inmost nature, is the product of the Divine Mind imaging forth an image of itself on the plane of the relative as the complementary to its own sphere of the absolute.

If we will therefore go to the *inmost* principle in ourselves, which philosophy and Scripture alike declare to be made in the image and likeness of God, instead of to the outer vehicles which it externalizes as instruments through which to function on the various planes of being, we shall find that we have reached a principle in ourselves which stands in *loco dei* towards all our vehicles and also towards our environment. It is above them all, and creates them, however unaware we may be of the fact, and relatively to them it occupies the place of first cause. The recognition of this is the discovery of our own relation to the whole world of the relative. On the other hand this must not lead us into the mistake of supposing that there is nothing higher, for, as we have already seen, this inmost principle or *ego* is itself the effect of an antecedent cause, for it proceeds from the imaging process in the Divine Mind.

We thus find ourselves holding an intermediate position between true First Cause, on the one hand, and the world of secondary causes on the other, and in order to understand the nature of this position, we must fall back on the axiom that the Universal can only work on the plane of the Particular through the individual. Then we see that the function of the individual is to *differentiate* the undistributed flow of the Universal into suitable directions for starting different trains of secondary causation.

Man's place in the cosmic order is that of a distributor of the Divine power, subject, however, to the inherent Law of the power which he distributes. We see one instance of this in ordinary science, in the fact that we never create force; all we can do is to distribute it. The very word Man means distributor or measurer, as in common with all words derived from the Sanderit root MN., it implies the idea of measurement, just as in the words moon, month, mens, mind, and " man," the Indian weight of 80lbs.; and it is for this reason that man is spoken of in Scripture as a " steward," or dispenser of the Divine gifts. As our minds become open to the full meaning of this position, the immense possibilities and also the responsibility contained in it will become apparent.

It means that the individual is the creative centre of his own world. Our past experience affords no evidence against this, but on the contrary, is evidence for it. Our true nature is always present, only we have hitherto taken the lower and mechanical side of things for our starting point, and so have created limitation instead of expansion. And even with the knowledge of the Creative Law which we have now attained, we shall continue to do this, if we seek our starting point in the things which are below us and not in the only thing which is above us, namely the Divine Mind, because it is only there that we can find illimitable Creative Power. Life is *being*, it is the experience of states of consciousness, and there is an unfailing correspondence between these inner states and our outward conditions. Now we see from the Original Creation that the state of consciousness must be the cause, and the corresponding conditions the effect, because at the starting of the creation no conditions existed, and the working of the Creative Mind upon itself can only have been a state of consciousness. This, then, is clearly the Creative Order—from states to conditions. But we invert this order, and seek to create from conditions to states. We say, If I had such and such conditions they would produce the state of feeling which I desire; and in so saying we run the risk of making a mistake as to the correspondence, for it may turn out that the particular conditions which we fixed on are not such as would produce the desired state. Or, again, though they might produce it in a certain degree, other conditions might produce it in a still greater degree, while at the same time opening the way to the attainment of still higher states and still better conditions. Therefore our wisest plan is to follow the pattern of the Parent Mind and make mental self-recognition our starting point, knowing that by the inherent Law of Spirit the corelated conditions will come by a natural process of growth. Then the great self-recognition is that of our relation to the Supreme Mind. That is the generating centre and we are distributing centres; just as electricity is generated at the central station and delivered in different forms of power by reason of passing through appropriate centres of distribution, so that in one place it lights a room, in another conveys a message, and in a third drives a tram car.   In like manner the power of the Universal Mind takes particular forms through the particular mind of the individual.   It does not interfere with the lines of his individuality, but works along them, thus making him, not less, but more himself.   It is thus, not a compelling power, but an expanding and illuminating one; so that the more the individual recognizes the reciprocal action between it and himself, the more full of life he must become.

Then also we need not be troubled about future conditions because we know that the All-originating Power is working through us and for us, and that according to the Law proved by the whole existing creation, it produces all the conditions required for the expression of the Life, Love and Beauty which it is, so that we can fully trust it to open the way as we go along.   The Great Teacher's words, "Take no thought for the morrow"—and note that the correct translation is "Take no anxious thought"—are the practical application of the soundest philosophy.   This does not, of course, mean that we are not to exert ourselves.   We must do our share in the work, and not expect God to do *for* us what He can only do *through* us.   We are to use our common sense and natural faculties in working upon the conditions now present.   We must make use of them, *as far as they go*, but we must not try and go further than the present things require; we must not try to force things, but allow them to grow naturally, knowing that they are doing so under the guidance of the All-Creating Wisdom.

Following this method we shall grow more and more into the habit of looking to mental attitude as the Key to our progress in Life, knowing that everything else must come out of that; and we shall further discover that our mental attitude is eventually determined by the way in which we regard the Divine Mind. Then the final result will be that we shall see the Divine Mind to be nothing else than Life, Love and Beauty—Beauty being identical with Wisdom or the perfect adjustment of parts to whole—and we shall see ourselves to be distributing centres of these primary energies and so in our turn subordinate centres of creative power. And as we advance in this knowledge we shall find that we transcend one law of limitation after another by finding the higher law, of which the lower is but a partial expression, until we shall see clearly before us, as our ultimate goal, nothing less than the Perfect Law of Liberty—not liberty without Law which is anarchy, but Liberty according to Law. In this way we shall find that the Apostle spoke the literal truth, when he said, that we shall become like Him when we see Him *as He is*, because the whole process by which our individuality is produced is one of reflection of the image existing in the Divine Mind. When we thus learn the Law of our own being we shall be able to specialize it in ways of which we have hitherto but little conception, but as in the case of all natural laws the specialization cannot take place until the fundamental principle of the generic law has been fully realized. For these reasons the student should endeavour to realize more and more perfectly, both in theory and practice, the law of the relation between the Universal and the Individual Minds. It is that of *reciprocal* action. If this fact of reciprocity is grasped, it will be found to explain both why the individual falls short of expressing the fulness of Life, which the Spirit is, and why he can attain to the fulness of that expression; just as the same law explains why iron sinks in water, and how it can be made to float. It is the individualizing of the Universal Spirit, by recognizing its reciprocity to ourselves, that is the secret of the perpetuation and growth of our own individuality.

THE NEW THOUGHT AND THE NEW ORDER.

In the two preceding lectures I have endeavoured to reach some conception of what the All-originating Spirit is in itself, and of the relation of the individual to it. So far as we can form any conception of these things at all we see that they are universal principles applicable to all nature, and, at the human level, applicable to all men: they are general laws the recognition of which is an essential preliminary to any further advance, because progress is made, not by setting aside the inherent law of things, which is impossible, but by specializing it through presenting conditions which will enable the same principle to act in a less limited manner. Having therefore got a general idea of these two ultimates, the universal and the individual, and of their relation to one another, let us now consider the process of specialization. In what does the specialization of a natural law consist? It consists in making that law or principle produce an effect which it could not produce under the simply generic conditions spontaneously provided by nature.

This selection of suitable conditions is the work of Intelligence, it is a process of consciously arranging things in a new order, so as to produce a new result. The principle is never new, for principles are eternal and universal; but the knowledge that the same principle will produce new results when working under new conditions is the key to the unfoldment of infinite possibilities. What we have therefore to consider is the working of Intelligence in providing specific conditions for the operation of universal principles, so as to bring about new results which will transcend our past experiences. The process does not consist in the introduction of new elements, but in making new combinations of elements which are always present; just as our ancestors had no conception of carriages that could go without horses, and yet by a suitable combination of elements which were always in existence, such vehicles are common objects in our streets to-day. How, then, is the power of Intelligence to be brought to bear upon the generic law of the relation between the Individual and the Universal so as to specialize it into the production of greater results than those which we have hitherto obtained?

All the practical attainments of science, which place the civilized world of to-day in advance of the times of King Alfred or Charlemagne, have been gained by a uniform method, and that a very simple one. It is by always enquiring what is the affirmative factor in any existing combination, and asking ourselves why, in that particular combination, it does not act beyond certain limits. What makes the thing a success, so far as it goes, and what prevents it going further? Then, by carefully considering the nature of the affirmative factor, we see what sort of conditions to provide to enable it to express itself more fully. This is the scientific method; it has proved itself true in respect of material things, and there is no reason why it should not be equally reliable in respect of spiritual things also.

Taking this as our method, we ask, What is the affirmative factor in the whole creation, and in ourselves as included in the creation, and, as we found in the first lecture, this factor is Spirit—that invisible power which concentrates the primordial ether into forms, and endows those forms with various modes of motion, from the simply mechanical motion of the planet up to the volitional motion in man. And, since this is so, the primary affirmative factor can only be the Feeling and the Thought of the Universal Spirit.* Now, by the hypothesis of the case, the Universal Spirit must be the Pure Essence of Life, and therefore its feeling and

---

* See my " Edinburgh Lectures on Mental Science."

thought can only be towards the continually increasing expression of the livingness which it is; and accordingly the specialization, of which we are in search, must be along the line of affording it a centre from which it may more perfectly realize this feeling and express this thought: in other words the way to specialize the generic principle of Spirit is by providing new mental conditions in consonance with its own original nature.

The scientific method of enquiry therefore brings us to the conclusion that the required conditions for translating the racial or generic operation of the Spirit into a specialized individual operation is a new way of *thinking*—a mode of thought concurring with, and not in opposition to, the essential forward movement of the Creative Spirit itself. This implies an entire reversal of our old conceptions. Hitherto we have taken forms and conditions as the starting point of our thought and inferred that *they* are the causes of mental states; now we have learnt that the true order of the creative process is exactly the reverse, and that thought and feeling are the causes, and forms and conditions the effects. When we have learnt this lesson we have grasped the foundation principle on which individual specialization of the generic law of the creative process becomes a practical possibility.

New Thought, then, is not the name of a particular sect, but is the essential factor by which our own future development is to be carried on; and its essence consists in seeing the relation of things in a New Order. Hitherto we have inverted the true order of cause and effect; now, by carefully considering the real nature of the Principle of Causation in itself—*causa causans* as distinguished from *causa causata*—we return to the true order and adopt a new method of thinking in accordance with it.

In themselves this order and this method of thinking are not new. They are older than the foundation of the world, for they are those of the Creative Spirit itself; and all through the ages this teaching has been handed down under various forms, the true meaning of which has been perceived only by a few in each generation. But as the light breaks in upon any individual it is a new light to him, and so to each one in succession it becomes the New Thought. And when anyone reaches it, he finds himself in a New Order. He continues indeed to be included in the universal order of the cosmos, but in a perfectly different way to what he had previously supposed; for, from his new standpoint, he finds that he is included, not so much as a part of the general effect, but as a part of the general cause; and when he perceives this he then sees that the method of his further advance must be by letting the General Cause flow more and more freely into his own specific centre, and he therefore seeks to provide thought conditions which will enable him to do so.

Then, still employing the scientific method of following up the affirmative factor, he realizes that this universal causative power, by whatever name he may call it, manifests as Supreme Intelligence in the adaptation of means to ends. It does so in the mechanism of the planet, in the production of supply for the support of physical life, and in the maintenance of the race as a whole. True, the investigator is met at every turn with individual failure; but his answer to this is that there is no cosmic failure, and that the apparent individual failure is itself a part of the cosmic process, and will diminish in proportion as the individual attains to the recognition of the Moving Principle of that process, and provides the necessary conditions to enable it to take a new starting point in his own individuality. Now, one of these conditions is to recognize it as Intelligence, and to remember that when working through our own mentality it in no way changes its essential nature, just as electricity loses none of its essential qualities in passing through the special apparatus which enables it to manifest as light.

When we see this, our line of thought will run something as follows:—" My mind is a centre of

Divine operation. The Divine operation is always for expansion and fuller expression, and this means the production of something beyond what has gone before, something entirely new, not included in past experience, though proceeding out of it by an orderly sequence of growth. Therefore, since the Divine cannot change its inherent nature, it must operate in the same manner in me; consequently in my own special world, of which I am the centre, it will move forward to produce new conditions, always in advance of any that have gone before." This is a legitimate line of argument, from the premises established in the recognition of the relation between the individual and the Universal Mind; and it results in our looking to the Divine Mind, not only as creative, but also as directive— that is as determining the actual forms which the conditions for its manifestation will take in our own particular world, as well as supplying the energy for their production. We miss the point of the relation between the individual and the universal, if we do not see that the Originating Spirit is a *forming* power. It is the forming power throughout nature, and if we would specialize it we must learn to trust its formative quality when operating from its new starting point in ourselves.

But the question naturally arises, If this is so, what part is taken by the individual? Our part is to provide a concrete centre round which the Divine energies can play. In the generic order of being we exercise upon it a force of attraction in accordance with the innate pattern of our particular individuality; and as we begin to realize the Law of this relation, we, in our turn, are attracted towards the Divine along the lines of least resistance, that is on those lines which are most natural to our special bent of mind. In this way we throw out certain aspirations with the result that we intensify our attraction of the Divine forces in a certain specific manner, and they then begin to act both through us and around us in accordance with our aspirations. This is the rationale of the reciprocal action between the Universal Mind and the individual mind, and this shows us that our desires should not be directed so much to the acquisition of particular *things* as to the reproduction in ourselves of particular phases of the Spirit's activity; and this, being in its very nature creative, is bound to externalize as corresponding things and circumstances. Then, when these external facts appear in the circle of our objective life, we must work upon them from the objective stand-point. This is where many fall short of completed work. They realize the subjective or creative process, but do not see that it must be followed by an objective or constructive process, and consequently they are unpractical dreamers and never reach the stage of completed work. The creative process brings the materials and conditions for the work to our hands; then we must make use of them with diligence and common-sense—God will provide the food, but He will not cook the dinner.

This, then, is the part taken by the individual, and it is thus that he becomes a distributing centre of the Divine energy, neither on the one hand trying to lead it like a blind force, nor on the other being himself under a blind unreasoning impulsion from it. He receives guidance because he seeks guidance; and he both seeks and receives according to a Law which he is able to recognize; so that he no more sacrifices his liberty or dwarfs his powers, than does an engineer who submits to the generic laws of electricity, in order to apply them to some specific purpose. The more intimate his knowledge of this Law of Reciprocity becomes, the more he finds that it leads on to Liberty, on the same principle by which we find in physical science that nature obeys us precisely in the same degree to which we first obey nature. As the esoteric maxim has it " What is a truth on one plane is a truth on all." But the key to this enfranchisement of body, mind, and circumstances is in that new thought which becomes creative of new conditions, because it realizes the true order of the creative process.

Therefore it is that, if we would bring a new order of Life, Light, and Liberty into our lives we must commence by bringing a new order into our thought, and find in ourselves the starting point of a new creative series, not by the force of personal will, but by union with the Divine Spirit, which in the expression of its inherent Love and Beauty, makes all things new.

THE LIFE OF THE SPIRIT.

THE three preceding lectures have touched upon certain fundamental truths in a definite order—first the nature of the Originating Spirit itself, next the generic relation of the individual to this All-embracing Spirit, and lastly the way to specialize this relation so as to obtain greater results from it than spontaneously arise by its merely generic action, and we have found that this can only be done through a new order of thought. This sequence is logical because it implies a Power, an Individual who understands the Power, and a Method of applying the power deduced from understanding its nature. These are general principles without realizing which it is impossible to proceed further, but assuming that the reader has grasped their significance, we may now go on to consider their application in greater detail.

Now this application must be a personal one, for it is only through the individual that the higher specialization of the power can take place, but at the same time this must not lead us to suppose that the individual, himself, brings the creative force into being. To suppose this is inversion; and we cannot impress upon ourselves too deeply that the relation of the individual to the Divine Spirit is that of a distributor, and not that of the original creator. If this is steadily borne in mind the way will become clear, otherwise we shall be led into confusion.

What, then, is the Power which we are to distribute? It is the Originating Spirit itself. We are sure that it is this because the new order of thought always begins at the beginning of any series which it contemplates bringing into manifestation, and it is based upon the fact that the origin of everything is Spirit. It is in this that its creative power resides; hence the person who is in the true new order of thought assumes as an axiomatic fact that what he has to distribute, or differentiate into manifestation is nothing else than the Originating Spirit. This being the case, it is evident that the *purpose* of the distribution must be the more perfect expression of the Originating Spirit as that which it is in itself, and what it is in itself is emphatically Life. What is seeking for expression, then, is the perfect Livingness of the Spirit; and this expression is to be found, through ourselves, by means of our renewed mode of thought. Let us see, then, how our new order of thought, with regard to the Principle of Life, is likely to operate.

In our old order of thought we have always associated Life with the physical body—life has been
for us the supreme physical fact. Now, however,
we know that Life is much more than this; but, as
the greater includes the less, it includes physical
life as one mode of its manifestation. The true
order does not require us to deny the reality of
physical life or to call it an illusion; on the contrary
it sees in physical life the completion of a great creative series, but it assigns it the proper place in that
series, which is what the old mode of thought did
not.

When we realize the truth about the Creative
Process, we see that the originating life is not
physical: its livingness consists in thought and feeling. By this inner movement it throws out vehicles through which to function, and these become
living forms because of the inner principle which
is sustaining them; so that the Life with which we
are primarily concerned in the new order is the
life of thought and feeling in ourselves as the vehicle, or distributing medium, of the Life of the
Spirit.

Then, if we have grasped the idea of the Spirit
as the great *forming* Power, as stated in the last
lecture, we shall seek in it the fountain-head of
Form as well as of Power: and as a logical deduction from this we shall look to it to give form to our

thoughts and feelings. If the principle is once recognised the sequence is obvious. The form taken by our outward conditions, whether of body or circumstance, depends on the form taken by our thoughts and feelings, and our thoughts and feelings will take form from that source from which we allow them to receive suggestion. Accordingly if we allow them to accept their fundamental suggestions from the relative and limited, they will assume a corresponding form and transmit them to our external environment, thus repeating the old order of limitation in a ceaselessly recurring round. Now our object is to get out of this circle of limitation, and the only way to do so is to get our thoughts and feelings moulded into new forms continually advancing to greater and greater perfection. To meet this requirement, therefore, there must be a forming power greater than that of our own unaided conceptions, and this is to be found in our realization of the Spirit as the Supreme Beauty, or Wisdom, moulding our thoughts and feelings into shapes harmoniously adjusted to the fullest expression, in and through us, of the Livingness which Spirit is in itself.

Now this is nothing more than transferring to the innermost plane of origination, a principle with which all readers who are " in the thought " may be presumed to be quite familiar—the principle of

Receptiveness. We all know what is meant by a receptive mental attitude when applied to healing or telepathy; and does it not logically follow that the same principle may be applied to the receiving of life itself from the Supreme Source? What is wanted, therefore, is to place ourselves in a receptive mental attitude towards the Universal Spirit with the intention of receiving its forming influence into our mental substance. It is always the presence of a definite intention that distinguishes the intelligent receptive attitude of mind from a merely sponge-like absorbancy, which sucks in any and every influence that may happen to be floating round: for we must not shut our eyes to the fact that there are various influences in the mental atmosphere by which we are surrounded, and some of them of the most undesirable kind. Clear and definite intention is therefore as necessary in our receptive attitude as in our active and creative one; and if our intention is to have our own thoughts and feelings moulded into such forms as to express those of the Spirit, then we establish that relation to the Spirit which, by the conditions of the case, must necessarily lead us to the conception of new ideals vitalised by a power which will enable us to bring them into concrete manifestation. It is in this way that we become differentiating centres of the Divine Thought giving it expression in form in the world of space and time, and thus is solved the great problem of enabling the Universal to act upon the plane of the particular without being hampered by those limitations which the merely generic law of manifestation imposes upon it. It is just here that subconscious mind performs the function of a " bridge " between the finite and the infinite as noted in my " Edinburgh Lectures on Mental Science " (page 31), and it is for this reason that a recognition of its susceptibility to impression is so important.

By establishing, then, a personal relation to the life of the Spirit, the sphere of the individual becomes enlarged. The reason is that he allows a greater intelligence than his own to take the initiative; and since he knows that this Intelligence is also the very Principle of Life itself, he cannot have any fear that it will act in any way to the diminution of his individual life, for that would be to stultify its own operation—it would be self-destructive action which is a contradiction in terms to the conception of Creative Spirit. Knowing, then, that by its inherent nature this Intelligence can only work to the expansion of the individual life, we can rest upon it with the utmost confidence and trust it to take an initiative which will lead to far greater results than any we could forecast from the stand-point of our own knowledge. So long as we insist on dictating the particular form which the action of the Spirit is to take, we limit it, and so close against ourselves avenues of expansion which might otherwise have been open to us; and if we ask ourselves why we do this we shall find that in the last resort it is because we do not believe in the Spirit as a *forming* power. We have, indeed, advanced to the conception of it as executive power, which will work to a prescribed pattern, but we have yet to grasp the conception of it as versed in the art of design, and capable of elaborating schemes of construction, which will not only be complete in themselves, but also in perfect harmony with one another. When we advance to the conception of the Spirit as containing in itself the ideal of Form as well as of Power, we shall cease from the effort of trying to force things into a particular shape, whether on the inner or the outer plane, and shall be content to trust the inherent harmoniousness or Beauty of the Spirit to produce combinations far in advance of anything that we could have conceived ourselves. This does not mean that we shall reduce ourselves to a condition of apathy, in which all desire, expectation and enthusiasm have been quenched, for these are the mainspring of our mental machinery; but on the contrary their action will be quickened by the knowledge that there is working at the back of

them a Formative Principle so infallible that it cannot miss its mark; so that however good and beau-
tiful the existing forms may be, we may always rest
in the happy expectation of something still better
to come. And it will come by a natural law of
growth, because the Spirit is in itself the Principle
of Increase. They will grow out of present conditions for the simple reason that if you are to reach
some further point it can only be by starting from
where you are now. Therefore it is written, " Des-
pise not the day of small things." There is only
one proviso attached to this forward movement of
the Spirit in the world of our own surroundings,
and that is that we shall co-operate with it; and
this co-operation consists in making the best use
of existing conditions in cheerful reliance on the
Spirit of Increase to express itself through us, and
for us, because we are in harmony with it. This
mental attitude will be found of immense value
in setting us free from worry and anxiety,
and as a consequence our work will be done
in a much more efficient manner. We shall
do the present work *for its own sake*, knowing
that herein is the principle of unfoldment; and doing it simply for its own sake we shall bring to
bear upon it a power of concentration which cannot fail of good results—and this quite naturally
and without any toilsome effort. We shall then

find that the secret of co-operation is to have faith in ourselves because we first have faith in God; and we shall discover that this Divine self-confidence is something very different from a boastful egotism which assumes a personal superiority over others. It is simply the assurance of a man who knows that he is working in accordance with a law of nature. He does not claim as a personal achievement what the Law does *for* him: but on the other hand he does not trouble himself about outcries against his presumptuous audacity raised by persons who are ignorant of the Law which he is employing. He is therefore neither boastful nor timorous, but simply works on in cheerful expectancy because he knows that his reliance is upon a Law which cannot be broken.

In this way, then, we must realize the Life of the Spirit as being also the Law of the Spirit. The two are identical, and cannot deny themselves. Our recognition of them gives them a new starting point through our own mentality, but they still continue to be the same in their nature, and unless limited or inverted by our mental affirmation of limited or inverted conditions, they are bound to work out into fuller and continually fuller expression of the Life, Love, and Beauty which the Spirit is in itself. Our path, therefore, is plain; it is simply to contemplate the Life, Love, and Beauty of the Originating Spirit and affirm that we are already giving expression to it in our thoughts and in our actions however insignificant they may at present appear. This path may be very narrow and humble in its beginning, but it ever grows wider and mounts higher, for it is the continually expanding expression of the Life of the Spirit which is infinite and knows no limits.

ALPHA AND OMEGA.

ALPHA and Omega, the First and the Last. What does this mean? It means the entire series of causation from the first originating movement to the final and completed result. We may take this on any scale from the creation of a cosmos to the creation of a lady's robe. Everything has its origin in an idea, a thought; and it has its completion in the manifestation of that thought in form. Many intermediate stages are necessary, but the Alpha and Omega of the series are the thought and the thing. This shows us that in essence the thing already existed in the thought. Omega is already potential in Alpha, just as in the Pythagorean system all numbers are said to proceed from unity and to be resolvable back again into it. Now it is this general principle of the already existence of the thing in the thought that we have to lay hold of, and as we find it true in an architect's design of the house that is to be, so we find it true in the great work of the Architect of the Universe. When we see this we have realized a general principle, which we find at work everywhere. That is the meaning of a *general* principle: it can be applied to any sort of subject; and the use of studying general principles is to give them particular application to anything we may have to deal with. Now what we have to deal with most of all is ourselves, and so we come to the consideration of Alpha and Omega in the human being. In the vision of St. John, the speaker of the words, "I am Alpha and Omega, the First and the Last," is described as " Like unto a son of man "—that is, however transcendent the appearance in the vision, it is essentially human, and thus suggests to us the presence of the universal principle at the human level. But the figure in the apocalyptic vision is not that of man as we ordinarily know him. It is that of Omega as it subsists enshrined in Alpha: it is the ideal of humanity as it subsists in the Divine Mind which was manifested in objective form to the eyes of the seer, and therefore presented the Alpha and Omega of that idea in all the majesty of Divine glory.

But if we grasp the truth that the thing is already existent in the thought, do we not see that this transcendent Omega must be already existent in the Divine ideal of every one of us? If on the plane of the absolute time is not, then does it not follow that this glorified humanity is a present fact in the Divine Mind? And if this is so, then this fact is eternally true regarding every human being. But if it is true that the thing exists in the thought, it is equally true that the thought finds form in the thing; and since things exist under the relative conditions of time and space, they are necessarily subject to a law of Growth, so that while the subsistence of the thing in the thought is perfect *ab initio*, the expression of the thought in the thing is a matter of gradual development. This is a point which we must never lose sight of in our studies; and we must never lose sight of the perfection of the thing in the thought because we do not yet see the perfection of the thought in the thing. Therefore we must remember that man, as we know him now, has by no means reached the ultimate of his evolution. We are only yet in the making, but we have now reached a point where we can facilitate the evolutionary process by conscious co-operation with the Creative Spirit. Our share in this work commences with the recognition of the Divine ideal of man, and thus finding the pattern by which we are to be guided. For since the person to be created after this pattern is ourself, it follows that, by whatever processes the Divine ideal transforms itself into concrete reality, the place where those processes are to work must be within ourselves; in other words, the creative action of the Spirit takes place through the laws of our own mentality. If it is a true maxim that the thing must take form in the thought before the thought can take form in the thing, then it is plain that the Divine Ideal can only be externalized in our objective life in proportion as it is first formed in our thought; and it takes form in our thought only to the extent to which we apprehend its existence in the Divine Mind. By the nature of the relation between the individual mind and the Universal Mind it is strictly a case of reflection; and in proportion as the mirror of our own mind blurs or clearly reflects the image of the Divine ideal, so will it give rise to a correspondingly feeble or vigorous reproduction of it in our external life.

This being the rationale of the matter, why should we limit our conception of the Divine ideal of ourselves? Why should we say, " I am too mean a creature ever to reflect so glorious an image "— or " God never intended such a limitless ideal to be reproduced in human beings." In saying such things we expose our ignorance of the whole Law of the Creative Process. We shut our eyes to the fact that the Omega of completion already subsists in the Alpha of conception, and that the Alpha of conception would be nothing but a lying illusion if it was not capable of expression in the Omega of completion. The creative process in us is that we become the individual reflection of what we realize

God to be relatively to ourselves, and therefore if we realize the Divine Spirit as the *infinite potential* of all that can constitute a perfected human being, this conception must, by the Law of the Creative Process, gradually build up a corresponding image in our mind, which in turn will act upon our external conditions.

This, by the laws of mind, is the nature of the process and it shows us what St. Paul means when he speaks of Christ being formed in us (Gal. iv. 19) and what in another place he calls being renewed in knowledge after the image of Him that created us (Col. iii. 10). It is a thoroughly logical sequence of cause and effect, and what we require is to see more clearly the Law of this sequence and use it intelligently—that is why St. Paul says it is being " renewed in knowledge ": it is a New Knowledge, the recognition of principles which we had not previously apprehended. Now the fact which, in our past experience, we have not grasped is that the human mind forms a new point of departure for the work of the Creative Spirit; and in proportion as we see this more and more clearly, the more we shall find ourselves entering into a new order of life in which we become less and less subject to the old limitations. This is not a reward arbitrarily bestowed upon us for holding dogmatically to certain mere verbal statements, but it is the natural result

of understanding the supreme law of our own being.   On its own plane it is as purely scientific as
the law of chemical re-action; only here we are not
dealing with the interaction of secondary causes
but with the Self-originating action of Spirit. Hence
a new force has to be taken into account which
does not occur in physical science, the power of
Feeling. Thought creates form, but it is feeling
that gives vitality to thought. Thought without
feeling may be constructive as in some great engi-
neering work, but it can never be creative as in the
work of the artist or musician; and that which originates within itself a new order of causation is, so
far as all pre-existing forms are concerned, a creation *ex nihilo*, and is therefore Thought expressive
of Feeling. It is this indissoluble union of
Thought and Feeling that distinguishes creative
thought from merely analytical thought and places
it in a different category; and therefore if we are to
afford a new starting-point for carrying on the work
of creation it must be by assimilating the feeling
of the Originating Spirit as part and parcel of its
thought—it is that entering into the Mind of the
Spirit of which I spoke in the first address.

Now the images in the Mind of the Spirit must
necessarily be *generic*. The reason for this is that
by its very nature the Principle of Life must be
prolific, that is, tending to Multiplicity, and there-

fore the original Thought-image must be fundamental to whole races, and not exclusive to particular individuals. Consequently the images in the Mind of the Spirit must be absolute types of the true essentials of the perfect development of the race, just what Plato meant by architypal ideas. This is the perfect subsistence of the thing in the thought. Therefore it is that our evolution as centres of *creative* activity, the exponents of new laws, and through them of new conditions, depends on our realizing in the Divine Mind the architype of mental perfection, at once as thought and feeling. But when we find all this in the Divine Mind, do we not meet with an infinite and glorious Personality? There is nothing lacking of all that we can understand by Personality, excepting outward form; and since the very essence of telepathy is that it dispenses with the physical presence, we find ourselves in a position of interior communion with a Personality at once Divine and Human. This is that Personality of the Spirit which St. John saw in the apocalyptic vision, and which by the very conditions of the case is the Alpha and Omega of Humanity.

But, as I have said, it is simply *generic* in itself, and it becomes active and specific only by a purely personal relation to the individual. But once more we must realize that nothing can take place except

according to Law, and therefore this specific relation is nothing arbitrary, but arises out of the generic Law applied under specific conditions. And
since what makes a law generic is precisely the
fact that it does not supply the specific conditions,
it follows that the conditions for the specialising of
the Law must be provided by the individual. Then
it is that his recognition of the originating creative
movement, as arising from combined Thought and
Feeling, becomes a practical working asset. He
realizes that there is a Heart and Mind of the
Spirit reciprocal to his own heart and mind, that he
is not dealing with a filmy abstraction, nor yet with
a mere mathematical sequence, but with something
that is pulsating with a Life as warm and vivid and
full of interest as his own—nay, more so, for it is
the Infinite of all that he himself is. And his recognition goes even further than this, for since this
specialization can only take place through the individual himself, it logically follows that the Life,
which he thus specializes, become *his own* life.
Quoad the individual it does not know itself apart
from him. But this self-recognition through the
individual cannot in any way change the inherent
nature of the Creative Spirit, and therefore to the
extent to which the individual perceives its identi-
fication with himself, he places himself under its
guidance, and so he becomes one of those who are

"led by the Spirit." Thus he begins to find the Alpha and Omega of the Divine ideal reproduced in himself—in a very small degree at present, but containing the principle of perpetual growth into an infinite expansion of which we can as yet form no conception.

St. John sums up the whole of this position in his memorable words:—" Beloved now are we the Sons of God, and it doth not yet appear what we *shall* be; but we know that when He shall appear (*i.e.*, become clear to us) we shall be like Him; for (*i.e.*, the reason of all this) we shall see Him as He is " (I. John iii. 2).

THE CREATIVE POWER OF THOUGHT.

ONE of the great axioms in the new order of ideas, of which I have spoken, is that our Thought possesses creative power, and since the whole superstructure depends on this foundation, it is well to examine it carefully. Now the starting point is to see that Thought, or purely mental action, is the only possible source from which the existing creation could ever have come into manifestation at all, and it is on this account that in the preceding addresses I have laid stress on the origin of the cosmos. It is therefore not necessary to go over this ground again, and we will start this morning's enquiry on the assumption that every manifestation is in essence the expression of a Divine Thought. This being so, our own mind is the expression of a Divine Thought. The Divine Thought has produced something which itself is capable of thinking; but the question is whether its thinking has the same creative quality as that of the Parent Mind.

Now by the very hypothesis of the case the whole Creative Process consists in the continual pressing forward of the Universal Spirit for expression through the individual and particular, and Spirit in its different modes is therefore the Life and Substance of the universe. Hence it follows that if there is to be an expression of thinking power it can only be by expressing the same thinking power which subsists latent in the Originating Spirit. If it were less than this it would only be some sort of mechanism and would not be thinking power, so that to be thinking power at all it must be identical in kind with that of the Originating Spirit. It is for this reason that man is said to be created in the image and likeness of God; and if we realize that it is impossible for him to be otherwise, we shall find a firm foundation from which to draw many important deductions.

But if our thought possesses this creative power, why are we hampered by adverse conditions? The answer is, because hitherto we have used our power invertedly. We have taken the starting point of our thought from external facts and consequently created a repetition of facts of a similar nature, and so long as we do this we must needs go on perpetuating the old circle of limitation. And, owing to the sensitiveness of the subconscious mind to suggestion—(See Edinburgh Lectures, chapter V.)—we are subject to a very powerful negative influence from those who are unacquainted with affirmative principles, and thus race-beliefs and the thought-currents of our more immediate environment tend to consolidate our own inverted thinking. It is therefore not surprising that the creative power of our thought, thus used in a wrong direction, has produced the limitations of which we complain. The remedy, then, is by reversing our method of thinking, and instead of taking external facts as our starting point, taking the inherent nature of mental power as our starting point. We have already gained two great steps in this direction, first by seeing that the whole manifested cosmos could have had its origin nowhere but in mental power, and secondly by realizing that our own mental power must be the same in kind with that of the Originating Mind.

Now we can go a step further and see how this power in ourselves can be perpetuated and intensified. By the nature of the creative process your mind is itself a thought of the Parent Mind; so, as long as this thought of the Universal Mind subsists, *you* will subsist, for you *are* it. But so long as you think this thought it continues to subsist, and necessarily remains present in the Divine Mind, thus fulfilling the logical conditions required for the perpetuation of the individual life. A poor analogy of the process may be found in a self-influencing dynamo where the magnetism generates the current and the current intensifies the magnetism with the result of producing a still stronger current until the limit of saturation is reached; only in the substantive infinitude of the Universal Mind and the potential infinitude of the Individual Mind there is no limit of saturation. Or we may compare the interaction of the two minds to two mirrors, a great and a small one, opposite each other, with the word " Life " engraved on the large one. Then, by the law of reflection, the word " Life " will also appear on the image of the smaller mirror reflected in the greater. Of course these are only very imperfect analogies; but if you can once grasp the idea of your own individuality as a thought in the Divine Mind which is able to perpetuate itself by thinking of itself as the thought which it is, you have got at the root of the whole matter, and by the same process you will not only perpetuate your life but will also expand it.

When we realize this on the one hand, and on the other that all external conditions, including the body, are produced by thought, we find ourselves standing between two infinites, the infinite of Mind and the infinite of Substance—from both of which we can draw what we will, and mould specific conditions out of the Universal Substance by the Creative Power which we draw in from the Universal Mind. But we must recollect that this is not by the force of personal will upon the substance, which is an error that will land us in all sorts of inversion, but by realizing our mind as a channel through which the Universal Mind operates upon substances in a particular way, according to the mode of thought which we are seeking to embody. If, then, our thought is habitually concentrated upon principles rather than on particular things, realizing that principles are nothing else than the Divine Mind in operation, we shall find that they will necessarily germinate to produce their own expression in corresponding facts, thus verifying the words of the Great Teacher, " Seek ye first the Kingdom of God and His righteousness and all these things shall be added unto you."

But we must never lose sight of the reason for the creative power of our thought, that it is because our mind is itself a thought of the Divine Mind, and that consequently our increase in livingness and creative power must be in exact proportion to our perception of our relation to the Parent Mind. In such considerations as these is to be found the philosophical basis of the Bible doctrine of " Sonship," with its culmination in the conception of the Christ. These are not mere fancies but the expression of strictly scientific principles, in their application to the deepest problems of the individual life; and their basis is that each one's world, whether in or out of the flesh, must necessarily be created by his own consciousness, and, in its turn, his mode of consciousness will necessarily take its colour from his conception of his relation to the Divine Mind—to the exclusion of light and colour, if he realizes no Divine Mind, and to their building up into forms of beauty in proportion as he realizes his identity of being with that All-Originating Spirit which is Light, Love, and Beauty in itself. Thus the great creative work of Thought in each of us is to make us consciously "sons and daughters of the Almighty," realizing that by our divine origin we can never be really separated from the Parent Mind which is continually seeking expression through us, and that any apparent separation is due to our own misconception of the true nature of the inherent relation between the Universal and the Individual. This is the lesson which the Great Teacher has so luminously put before us in the parable of the Prodigal Son.

THE GREAT AFFIRMATIVE.

THE Great Affirmative appears in two modes, the cosmic and the individual. In its essence it is the same in both, but in each it works from a different standpoint. It is always the principle of Being—that which *is*, as distinguished from that which is not; but to grasp the true significance of this saying we must understand what is meant by " that which is not." It is something more than mere non-existence, for obviously we should not trouble ourselves about what is non-existent. It is that which both is and is not at the same time, and the thing that answers to this description is " Conditions." The little affirmative is that which affirms particular conditions as all that it can grasp, while the great affirmative grasps a wider conception, the conception of that which gives rise to conditions. Cosmically it is that power of Spirit which sends forth the whole creation as its expression of itself, and it is for this reason that I have drawn attention in the preceding lectures to the idea of the creation *ex nihilo* of the whole visible universe. As Eastern and Western Scriptures alike tell us it is the breath-

ing-forth of Original Spirit; and if you have followed what I have said regarding the reproduction
of this Spirit in the individual—that by the very
nature of the creative process the human mind
must be of the same quality with the Divine Mind
—then we find that a second mode of the Originating Spirit becomes possible, namely that of operation through the individual mind. But whether
acting cosmically or personally it is always the
same Spirit and therefore cannot lose its inherent
character which is that of the Power which creates
ex nihilo. It is the direct contradiction of the
maxim " ex nihilo nihil fit "—nothing can be made
out of nothing; and it is the recognition of the
presence in ourselves of this power, which can make
something out of nothing, that is the key to our
further progress. As the logical outcome of the
cosmic creative process, the evolutionary work
reaches a point where the Originating Power creates an image of itself; and thus affords a fresh
point of departure from which it can work specifi-
cally, just as in the cosmic process it works gener-
ically. From this new standpoint it does not in
any way contradict the laws of the cosmic order,
but proceeds to specialize them, and thus to bring
out results through the individual which could not
be otherwise attained.

Now the Spirit does this by the same method as

in the Original Creation, namely by creating *ex nihilo;* for otherwise it would be bound by the limitations necessarily inherent in the cosmic *form* of things, and so no fresh creative starting point would have been attained. This is why the Bible lays such stress on the principle of Monogenesis, or creation from a single power instead of from a pair or syzegy; and it is on this account that we are told that this One-ness of God is the foundation of all the commandments, and that the " Son of God " is declared to be " monogenes " or one-begotten, for that is the correct translation of the Greek word. The immense importance of this principle of creation from a single power will become apparent as we realize more fully the results proceeding from the assumption of the opposite principle, or the dualism of the creative power; but as the discussion of this great subject would require a volume to itself, I must, at present, content myself with saying that this insistence of the Bible upon the singleness of the Creative Power is based upon a knowledge which goes to the very root of esoteric principles, and is therefore not to be set aside in favour of dualistic systems, though superficially the latter may appear more consonant to reason.

If, then, it is possible to put the Great Affirmation into words it is that God is ONE and that this ONE finds centre in ourselves; and if the full meaning of this statement is realized, the logical result will be found to be a new creation both in and from ourselves. We shall realize in ourselves the working of a new principle whose distinguishing feature is its simplicity. It is ONE-ness and is not troubled about any second. Hence what it contemplates is not how its action will be modified by that of some second principle, something which will compel it to work in a particular manner and so limit it; but what it contemplates is its own Unity. Then it perceives that its Unity consists in a greater and a lesser movement, just as the rotation of the earth on its axis does not interfere with its rotation round the sun but are both motions of the same unit, and are definitely related to each other. In like manner we find that the Spirit is moving simultaneously in the macrocosm of the universe and in the microcosm of the individual, and the two movements harmonize because they are that of the same Spirit, and the latter is included in the former and pre-supposes it. The Great Affirmation, therefore, is the perception that the " I AM " is ONE, always harmonious with itself, and including all things in this harmony for the simple reason that there is no second creative power; and when the individual realizes that this always-single power is the root of his own being, and therefore has centre in himself and finds expression through him, he

learns to trust its singleness and the consequent
harmony of its action *in* him with what it is doing
around him.   Then he sees that the affirmation " I
and my Father are ONE " is a necessary deduction
from a correct apprehension of the fundamental
principles of being; and then, on the principle that
the less must be included in the greater, he desires
that harmonious unity of action be maintained by
the adaptation of his own particular movement to
the larger movement of the Spirit working as the
Creative Principle through the great whole.   In
this way we become centres through which the creative forces find specialization by the development
of that personal factor on which the specific application of general laws must always depend.   A specific sort of individuality is formed, capable of being the link between the great Spiritual Power of
the universal and the manifestation of the relative
in time and space because it consciously partakes
of both; and because the individual of this class
recognizes the singleness of the Spirit as the starting point of all things, he endeavours to withdraw
his mind from all arguments derived from external
conditions, whether past or present, and to fix it
upon the forward movement of the Spirit which he
knows to be always identical both in the universe
and in himself.   He ceases the attempt to dictate
to the Spirit, because he does not see in it a mere

blind force, but reveres it as the Supreme Intelligence: and on the other hand he does not grovel before it in doubt and fear, because he knows it is one with himself and is realizing itself through him, and therefore cannot have any purpose antagonistic to his own individual welfare. Realizing this he deliberately places his thoughts under the guidance of the Divine Spirit, knowing that his outward acts and conditions must thereby be brought into harmony with the great forward movement of the Spirit, not only at the stage he has now reached, but at all future stages. He does not at all deny the power of his own thought as the creative agent in his own personal world,—on the contrary it is precisely on the knowledge of this fact that his perception of the true adjustment between the principles of Life is based; but for this very reason he is the more solicitous to be led by that Wisdom which can see what he cannot see, so that his personal control over the conditions of his own life may be employed to its continual increase and development.

In this way our affirmation of the " I am " ceases to be the petulant assertion of our limited personality and becomes the affirmation that the Great I AM affirms its own I AM-ness both in us and through us, and thus our use of the words becomes in very truth the Great Affirmative, or that which is the root of all being as distinguished from that which has no being in itself but is merely externalized by being as the vehicle for its expression. We shall realize our true place as subordinate creative centres, perfectly independent of existing conditions because the creative process is that of monogenesis and requires no other factor than the Spirit for its exercise, but at the same time subordinate to the Divine Spirit in the greatness of its inherent forward movement because there is only ONE Spirit and it cannot from one centre antagonize what it is doing from another. Thus the Great Affirmation makes us children of the Great King, at once living in obedience to that Power which is above us, and exercising this same power over all that world of secondary causation which is below us.

Thus in our measure and station each one of us will receive the mission of the I AM.

CHRIST THE FULFILLING OF THE LAW.

"Think not that I am come to destroy the law or the proph-
ets: I am not come to destroy but to fulfil." (Matt. v. 17.)
"Christ is the end of the law for righteousness to everyone
that believeth." (Rom. x. 4.)

IF these words are the utterance of a mere sec-
tarian superstition they are worthless; but if they
are the statement of a great principle, then it is
worth our while to enquire what that principle is.
The fulfilling of anything is the bringing into complete realization of all that it potentially contains,
and so the filling of any law to its fulness means
bringing out all the possibilities which are hidden
in it. This is precisely the method which has
brought forth all the advances of material civiliza-
tion. The laws of nature are the same now that
they were in the days of our rugged Anglo-Saxon
ancestors, but they brought out only an infinitesi-
mal fraction of the possibilities which those laws
contain : now we have brought out a good deal
more, but we have by no means exhausted them,
and so we continue to advance, not by contradict-
ing natural laws, but by more fully realizing their

63

capacity. Why should we not, then, apply the same method to ourselves and see whether there are no potentialities hidden away in the law of our own being which we have not as yet by any means brought to their fulfilment? We talk of a good time coming and of the ameliorating of the race; but do we reflect that the race is composed of individuals and that therefore real advance is to be made only by individual improvement, and not by Act of Parliament? and if so, then the individual with whom to begin is ourself.

The complete manifestation of the Law of Individuality is the end or purpose of the Bible teaching concerning Christ. It is a teaching based upon Law, spiritual and mental, fully recognizing that no effect can be produced except by the operation of an adequate cause; and Christ is set before us both as explaining the causes and exhibiting the full measure of the effects. All this is according to Law; and the importance of its being according to Law is that Law is universal, and the potentialities of the Law are therefore inherent in everyone—there is no special law for anybody, but anybody can specialize the law by using it with a fuller understanding of how much can be got out of it; and the purpose of the Scripture teaching regarding Christ is to help us to do this.

The preceding lectures have led us step by step

to see that the Originating Spirit, which first brought the world into existence, is also the root of our own individuality, and is therefore always ready, by its inherent nature, to continue the creative process from this individual stand-point as soon as the necessary conditions are provided, and these conditions are thought-conditions. Then by realizing the relation of Christ to the Originating Mind, the Parent Spirit or " Father," we receive a *standard* of thought which is bound to act creatively bringing out all the potentialities of our hidden being. Now the relation of Christ to the " Father " is that of the Architypal Idea in the All-creating Mind of which I have previously spoken, and so we arrive at the conception of the Christ-idea as a universal principle, and as being an idea therefore capable of reproduction in the individual Mind, thus explaining St. Paul's meaning when he speaks of Christ being formed in us. It is here that the principle of monogenesis comes in, that principle which I have endeavoured to describe in the earlier part of the present series as originating the whole manifested creation by an internal action of the Spirit upon itself; and it is the entire absence of control by any second power that renders the realization in external actuality of a purely mental ideal possible. For this reason systematic spiritual study commences with the contemplation of the existing cosmos, and we then transfer the conception of the monogenetic power of the Spirit from the cosmos to the individual and realize that the same Spirit is able to do the same thing in ourselves. This is the New Thought which in time will fulfil itself in the New Order, and we thus provide new thought-conditions which enable the Spirit to carry on its creative work from a new stand-point, that of our own individuality. This attainment by the Spirit of a new starting-point is what is meant by the esoteric doctrine of the Octave. The Octave is the starting-point of a new series reduplicating the starting-point of the previous series at a different level, just as does the octave note in music. We find this principle constantly referred to in Scripture—the completion of a prior series in the number Seven, and the starting of a new series by the number Eight, which takes the same place in the second series that the number One did in the first. The second series comes out of the first by natural growth and could not come into existence without it, hence the First or Originating number of the second series is the Eighth if we regard the second series as the prolongation of the first. Seven is the numerical correspondence of complete manifestation because it is the combination of three and four, which respectively represent the complete working of the spiritual and material factors—involution and evolution—and thus together constitute the finished whole. Students of the Tarot will here realize the process by which the Yod of Yod becomes the Yod of He. It is for this reason that the primary or cosmic creation terminates in the rest of the Seventh Day, for it can proceed no further until a fresh starting-point is found. But when this fresh starting-point is found in Man realizing his relation to the " Father," we start a new series and strike the Creative Octave and therefore the Resurrection takes place, not on the Sabbath or Seventh Day, but on the Eighth day which then becomes the First day of the new creative week. The *principle* of the Resurrection is the realization by man of his individualization of the Spirit and his recognition of the fact that, since the Spirit is always the same Spirit, it becomes the Alpha of a new creation from his own centre of being.

Now all this is necessarily an interior process taking place on the mental plane; but if we realize that the creative process is always primarily one of involution, or formation in the spiritual world, we shall grasp something of the meaning of Christ as " The Son of God "—the concentration of the Universal Spirit into a Personality on the spiritual plane correlatively to the individuality of each one who affords the necessary thought-conditions. To all who apprehend it there is then discovered in the

Universal Spirit the presence of a Divine Individuality reciprocal to that of the individual man, the
recognition of which is the practical solution of all
metaphysical problems regarding the emanation of
the individual soul from the Universal Spirit and
the relations arising therefrom; for it takes these
matters out of the region of intellectual speculation,
which is never creative but only analytical, and
transfers it to the region of feeling and spiritual
sensation which is the abode of the creative forces.
This personal recognition of the Divine then affords us a new basis of Affirmation, and we need no
longer trouble to go further back in order to an-
alyze it, because we know experimentally that it
is there; so now we find the starting-point of the
new creation ready-made for us according to the
architypal pattern in the Divine Mind itself and
therefore perfectly correctly formed. When once
this truth is clearly apprehended, whether we reach
it by an intellectual process or by simple intuition,
we can make it our starting-point and claim to have
our thought permeated by the creative power of
the Spirit on this basis.

But vast as is the conception thus reached we
must remember that it is still a starting-point. It,
indeed, transcends our previous range of ideas and
so presents a culmination of the cosmic creative
series which passes beyond that series and thus

brings us to number Eight or the Octave; but on this very account it is the number One of a new creative series which is personal to the individual.

Then, because the Spirit is always the same, we may look for a repetition of the creative process at a higher level, and, as we all know, that process consists first of the involution of Spirit into Substance, and consequently of the subsequent evolution of Substance into forms continually increasing in fitness as vehicles for Spirit: so now we may look for a repetition of this universal process from its new starting-point in the individual mind and expect a corresponding externalization in accordance with our familiar axiom that thoughts are things.

Now it is as such an external manifestation of the Divine ideal that the Christ of the Gospels is set before us. I do not wish to dogmatize, but I will only say that the more clearly we realize the nature of the creative process on the spiritual side the more the current objections to the Gospel narrative lose their force; and it appears to me that to deny that narrative as a point-blank impossibility is to make a similar affirmation with regard to the power of the Spirit in ourselves. You cannot affirm a principle and deny it in the same breath; and if we affirm the externalizing power of the Spirit in our own case, I do not see how we can logically lay down a limit for its action and say that under highly

specialized conditions it could not produce highly
specialized effects. It is for this reason that St.
John puts the question of Christ manifest in the
flesh as the criterion of the whole matter (I. John
iv., 2). If the Spirit can create at all then you cannot
logically limit the extent or method of its working;
and since the basis of our expectation of individual
expansion is the limitless creative power of the
Spirit, to reject the Christ of the Gospels as an impossibility is to cut away the ground from under our
own feet. It is one thing to say " I do not understand why the Spirit should have worked in that
way "—that is merely an honest statement of our
present stage of knowledge, or we may even go the
length of saying that we do not feel convinced that
it did work in that way—that is a true confession
of our intellectual difficulty—but certainly those
who are professedly relying on the power of the
Spirit to produce external results cannot say that
it does not possess that power, or possesses it only
in a limited degree: the position is logically self-destructive. What we should do therefore, is to sus-
pend judgment and follow the light as far as we can
see it, and bye-and-bye it will become clearer to us.
There are, it appears to me, occult heights in the
doctrine of Christ designed by the Supreme Wisdom to counteract corresponding occult depths in
the Mystery of Darkness. I do not think it is at

all necessary, or even possible, for us to scale these heights or fathom those depths, with our present infantile intelligence, but if we realize how completely the law of our being receives its fulfilment in Christ as far as we know that law, may we not well conceive that there are yet deeper phases of that law the existence of which we can only faintly surmise by intuition? Occasionally just the fringe of the veil is lifted for some of us, but that momentary glance is enough to show us that there are powers and mysteries beyond our present conception. But even there Law reigns supreme, and therefore taking Christ as our basis and starting-point, we start with the Law already fulfilled, whether in those things which are familiar to us or in those realms which are beyond our thought, and so we need have no fear of evil. Our starting-point is that of a divinely ordained security from which we may quietly grow into that higher evolution which is the fulfilment of the law of our own being.

THE STORY OF EDEN.

THE whole Bible and the whole history of the world, past, present and future, are contained in embryo in the story of Eden, for they are nothing else than the continuous unfolding of certain great principles which are there allegorically stated. That this is by no means a new notion is shown by the following quotation from Origen:—"Who is there so foolish and without common-sense as to believe that God planted trees in the Garden of Eden like a husbandman; and planted therein the tree of life perceptible to the eyes and to the senses, which gave life to the eater; and another tree which gave to the eater a knowledge of good and evil? I believe that everybody must regard these as figures under which a recondite sense is concealed." Let us, then, follow up the suggestion of this early Father of the Church, and enquire what may be the "recondite sense" concealed under this figure of the two trees. On the face of the story there are two roots, one of Life and the other of Death, two fundamental principles bringing about diametrically opposite results. The distinctive mark of the latter is that it is the knowledge of good and evil, that is to say, the recognition of two antagonistic principles, and so requiring a knowledge of the relations between them to enable us to continually make the needful adjustments to keep ourselves going. Now, in appearance this is exceedingly specious. It looks so entirely reasonable that we do not see its ultimate destructiveness; and so we are told that Eve ate the fruit because she " saw that the tree was pleasant to the eyes." But careful consideration will show us in what the destructive nature of this principle consists. It is based on the fallacy that good is limited by evil, and that you cannot receive any good except through eliminating the corresponding evil by realizing it and beating it back. In this view life becomes a continual combat against every imaginable form of evil, and after we have racked our brains to devise precautions against all possible evil happenings, there remains the chance, and much more than the chance, that we have by no means exhausted the category of negative possibilities, and that others may arise which no amount of foresight on our part could have imagined. The more we see into this position the more intolerable it becomes, because from this stand-point we can never attain any certain basis of action, and the forces of possible evil multiply as we contemplate them. To

set forth to out-wit all evil by our own knowledge
of its nature is to attempt a task the hopelessness
of which becomes apparent when we see it in its
true light.

The mistake is in supposing that Life can be
generated in ourselves by an intellectual process;
but, as we have seen in the preceding lectures, Life
is the primary movement of the Spirit, whether in
the cosmos or in the individual.   In its proper order
intellectual knowledge is exceedingly important and
useful, but its place in the order of the whole is
not that of the Originator.   It is not Life in itself,
but is a function of life; it is an effect and not the
cause.   The reason why this is so is because intellectual study is always the study of the various
laws which arise from the different *relations* of
things to one another; and it therefore presupposes
that these things together with their laws are already in existence.   Consequently it does not start
from the truly creative stand-point, that of creating
something entirely new, creation *ex nihilo* as distinguished from *construction*, or the laying-together
of existing materials, which is what the word literally means.   To recognize evil as a force to be
reckoned with is therefore to give up the creative
stand-point altogether.   It is to quit the plane of
First Cause and descend into the realm of secondary causation and lose ourselves amid the confusion

of a multiplicity of relative causes and effects without grasping any unifying principle behind them.

Now the only thing that can release us from the inextricable confusion of an infinite multiplicity is the realization of an underlying unity, and at the back of all things we find the presence of one Great Affirmative principle without which nothing could have existence. This, then, is the Root of Life; and if we credit it with being able, not only to supply the power, but also the form for its manifestation we shall see that we need not go beyond this *single* Power for the production of anything. It is Spirit producing Substance out of its own essence, and the Substance taking Form in accordance with the movement of the Spirit. What we have to realize is, not only that this is the way in which the cosmos is brought into existence, but also that, because the Spirit finds a new centre in ourselves, the same process is repeated in our own mentality, and therefore we are continually creating *ex nihilo* whether we know it or not. Consequently, if we look upon evil as a force to be reckoned with, and therefore requiring to be studied, we are in effect creating it; while on the other hand if we realize that there is only *one* force to be considered, and that absolutely good, we are by the law of the creative process bringing that good into manifestation. No doubt for this affirmative use of our creative power it is necessary that we start from the basic conception of a *single* originating power which is absolutely good and life-giving; but if there were a self-originating power which was destructive then no creation could ever have come into existence at all, for the positive and negative self-originating powers would cancel each other and the result would be zero. The fact, therefore, of our own existence is a sufficient proof of the singleness and goodness of the Originating Power, and from this starting-point there is no second power to be taken into consideration, and consequently we do not have to study the evil that may arise out of existing or future circumstances, but require to keep our minds fixed only upon the good which we intend to create. There is a very simple reason for this. It is that every new creation necessarily carries its own law with it and by that law produces new conditions of its own. A balloon affords a familiar illustration of my meaning. The balloon with its freight weighs several hundredweight, yet the introduction of a new factor, the gas, brings with it a law of its own which entirely alters the conditions, and the force of gravity is so completely overcome that the whole mass rises into the air. The Law itself is never altered, but we have previously known it only under limiting conditions. These conditions, however, are no part of the Law itself; and a clearer realization of the Law shows us that it contains in itself the power of transcending them. The law which every new creation carries with it is therefore not a contradiction of the old law but its specialization into a higher mode of action.

Now the ultimate Law is that of production *ex nihilo* by the movement of the Spirit within itself, and all subordinate laws are merely the measurements of the relations which spontaneously arise between different things when they are brought into manifestation, and therefore, if an entirely new thing is created it must necessarily establish entirely new relations and so produce entirely new laws. This is the reason why, if we take the action of pure unmanifested Spirit as our starting-point, we may confidently trust it to produce manifestations of law which, though perfectly new from the stand-point of our past experience, are quite as natural in their own way as any that have gone before. It is on this account that in these addresses I lay so much stress on the fact that Spirit creates *ex nihilo*, that is, out of no pre-existing forms, but simply by its own movement within itself. If, then, this idea is clearly grasped, it logically follows from it that the Root of Life is not to be found in the comparison of good and evil, but in the simple affirmation of the Spirit as the All-creating power of Good. And since, as we have

already seen, this same all-creating Spirit finds a
centre and fresh starting-point of operation in our
own minds, we can trust it to follow the Law of its
own being there as much as in the creation of the
cosmos.

Only we must not forget that it is working
through our own minds. It thinks through our
mind, and our mind must be made a suitable channel for this mode of its operation by conforming itself to the broad generic lines of the Spirit's
thinking. The reason for this is one which I have
sought to impress throughout these lectures, namely, that the specialization of a law is never the
denial of it, but on the contrary the fuller recognition of its basic principles; and if this is the case in
ordinary physical science it must be equally so when
we come to specialize the great Law of Life itself.
The Spirit can never change its essential nature as
the essence of Life, Love, and Beauty; and if we
adopt these characteristics, which constitute the
Law of the Spirit, as the basis of our own thinking,
and reject all that is contrary to them, then we
afford the broad generic conditions for the specialized thinking of the Spirit through our own minds:
and the thinking of the Spirit is that *involution*, or
passing of spirit into form, which is the whole being of the creative process.

The mind which is all the time being thus formed

is our own. It is not a case of control by an external individuality, but the fuller expression of the Universal through an organized mentality which has all along been a less perfect expression of the Universal; and therefore the process is one of growth. We are not losing our individuality, but are coming into fuller possession of ourselves by the conscious recognition of our personal share in the great work of creation. We begin in some slight measure to understand what the Bible means when it speaks of our being " partakers of the Divine nature " (II. Peter i. 4) and we realize the significance of the " unity of the Spirit " (Ephesians iv. 3). Doubtless this will imply changes in our old mode of thinking; but these changes are not forced upon us, they are brought about naturally by the new stand-point from which we now see things. Almost imperceptibly to ourselves we grow into a New Order of Thought which proceeds, not from a knowledge of good and evil, but from the Principle of Life itself. That is what makes the difference between our old thought and our new thought. Our old thought was based upon a comparison of limited facts: our new thought is based upon a comprehension of principles. The difference is like that between the mathematics of the infant, who cannot count beyond the number of apples or marbles put before him, and that of the

senior wrangler who is not dependent upon visible
objects for his calculations, but plunges boldly into
the unknown because he knows that he is working
by indubitable principles.　In like manner when we
realize the infallible Principle of the Creative Law
we no longer find we need to see everything cut
and dried beforehand, for if so, we could never get
beyond the range of our old experiences; but we
can move steadily forward because we know the
certainty of the creative principle by which we are
working, or rather, which is working through us,
and that our life, in all its minutest details, is its
harmonious expression.　Thus the Spirit thinks
through our thought only its thought is greater
than ours.　It is the paradox of the less containing
the greater.　Our thought will not be objectless or
unintelligible to ourselves.　It will be quite clear
as far as it goes.　We shall know exactly what we
want to do and why we want to do it, and so will
act in a reasonable and intelligent manner.　But
what we do not know is the greater thought that
is all the time giving rise to our smaller thought,
and which will open out from it as our lesser
thought progresses into form.　Then we gradually
see the greater thought which prompted our smaller one and we find ourselves working along its
lines, guided by the invisible hand of the Creative
Spirit into continually increasing degrees of living-

ness to which we need assign no limits, for it is the expansion of the Infinite within ourselves.

This, as it appears to me, is the hidden meaning of the two trees in Eden, the Garden of the Soul. It is the distinction between a knowledge which is merely that of comparisons between different sorts of conditions, and a knowledge which is that of the Life which gives rise to and therefore controls conditions. Only we must remember that the control of conditions is not to be attained by violent self-assertion which is only recognizing them as substantive entities to be battled with, but by conscious unity with that All-creating Spirit which works silently, but surely, on its own lines of Life, Love, and Beauty.

" Not by might, nor by power, but by My Spirit, saith the Lord of Hosts."

THE WORSHIP OF ISHI.

In Hosea ii. 16 we find this remarkable statement:—" And it shall be at that day, saith the Lord, that thou shalt call Me Ishi, and shalt no more call Me Baali "; and with this we may couple the statement in Isaiah lxii. 4:—" Thou shalt be called Hephzibah, and thy land Beulah; for the Lord delighteth in thee, and thy land shall be married."

In both these passages we find a change of name; and since a name stands for something which corresponds to it, and in truth only amounts to a succinct description, the fact indicated in these texts is a change of condition answering to the change of name.

Now the change from Baali to Ishi indicates an important alteration in the relation between the Divine Being and the worshipper; but since the Divine Being cannot change, the altered relation must result from a change in the stand-point of the worshipper: and this can only come from a new mode of looking at the Divine, that is, from a new order of thought regarding it. Baali means Lord, and Ishi means husband, and so the change in relation is that of a female slave who is liberated and married to her former master. We could not have a more perfect analogy. Relatively to the Universal Spirit the individual soul is esoterically feminine, as I have pointed out in " Bible Mystery and Bible Meaning," because its function is that of the receptive and formative. This is necessarily inherent in the nature of the creative process. But the individual's development as the specializing medium of the Universal Spirit will depend entirely upon his own conception of his relation to it. So long as he only regards it as an arbitrary power, a sort of slave owner, he will find himself in the position of a slave driven by an inscrutable force, he knows not whither or for what purpose. He may worship such a God, but his worship is only the worship of fear and ignorance, and there is no personal interest in the matter except to escape some dreaded punishment. Such a worshipper would gladly escape from his divinity, and his worship, when analyzed, will be found to be little else than disguised hatred. This is the natural result of a worship based upon *unexplained* traditions instead of intelligible principles, and is the very opposite of that worship in Spirit and in truth which Jesus speaks of as the true worship.

But when the light begins to break in upon us, all this becomes changed. We see that a system of terrorism cannot give expression to the Divine Spirit, and we realize the truth of St. Paul's words,

"He hath not given us the spirit of fear, but of power, and of love, and of a sound mind." As the true nature of the relation between the individual mind and the Universal Mind becomes clearer, we find it to be one of mutual action and re-action, a perfect reciprocity which cannot be better symbolized than by the relation between an affectionate husband and wife. Everything is done from love and nothing from compulsion, there is perfect confidence on both sides, and both are equally indispensable to each other. It is simply the carrying out of the fundamental maxim that the Universal cannot act on the plane of the Particular except through the Particular; only this philosophical axiom develops into a warm living intercourse.

Now this is the position of the soul which is indicated by the name Hephzibah. In common with all other words derived from the Semitic root " hafz " it implies the idea of guarding, just as in the East a *hafiz* is one who guards the letter of the Koran by having the whole book by heart, and in many similar expressions. Hephzibah may therefore be translated as " a guarded one," thus recalling the New Testament description of those who are " guarded into salvation." It is precisely this conception of being guarded by a superior power that distinguishes the worship of Ishi from that of Baali. A special relation has been established between the Divine Spirit and the individual soul, one of absolute confidence and personal intercourse. This does not require any departure from the general law of the universe, but is due to that specializing of the law through the presentation of special conditions personal to the individual, of which I have spoken before. But all the time there has been no change in the Universal Spirit, the only change has been in the mental attitude of the individual—he has come into a new thought, a clearer perception of God. He has faced the questions, What is God? Where is God? How does God work? and he has found the answer in the apostolic statement that God is " over all, through all, and in all," and he realises that " God " is the root of his (the individual's) own being, ever present *in* him, ever working *through* him, and universally present around him.

This realization of the true relation between the Originating Spirit and the individual mind is what is esoterically spoken of as the Mystical Marriage in which the two have ceased to be separate and have become one. As a matter of fact they always were one, but since we can apprehend things only from the stand-point of our own consciousness, it is our recognition of the fact that makes it a practical reality for ourselves. But an intelligent recognition will never make a confusion of the two parts of which the whole consists, and will never lead the individual to suppose that he is handling a blind force or that a blind force is handling him. He will neither dethrone God, nor lose himself by absorption in deity, but he will recognize the reciprocity of the Divine and the human as the natural and logical outcome of the essential conditions of the creative process.

And what is the Whole which is thus created? It is our conscious *personality ;* and therefore whatever we draw from the Universal Spirit acquires in us the quality of personality. It is that process of differentiation of the universal into the particular of which I have so often spoken, which, by a rude analogy, we may compare to the differentiation of the universal electric fluid into specific sorts of power by its passage through suitable apparatus. It is for this reason that relatively to ourselves the Universal Spirit must necessarily assume a personal aspect, and that the aspect which it will assume will be in exact correspondence with our own conception of it. This is in accordance with mental and spiritual laws inherent in our own being, and it is on this account that the Bible seeks to build up our conception of God on such lines as will set us free from all fear of evil, and thus leave us at liberty to use the creative power of our thought affirmatively from the stand-point of a calm and untroubled mind. This stand-point can only be reached by passing beyond the range of the happenings of the moment, and this can only be done by the discovery of our immediate relation to the undifferentiated source of all good. I lay stress on these words "immediate" and "undifferentiated" because in them is contained the secret of the whole position. If we could not draw immediately from the Universal Spirit our receiving would be subject to the limitations of the channel through which it reached us; and if the force which we receive were not undifferentiated in itself it could not take appropriate form in our own minds and become to each of us just what we require it to be. It is this power of the human soul to differentiate limitlessly from the Infinite that we are apt to overlook, but as we come to realize that the soul is itself a reflection and image of the Infinite Spirit—and a clear recognition of the cosmic creative process shows that it cannot be anything else—we find that it must possess this power, and that in fact it is our possession of this power which is the whole *raison d'etre* of the creative process: if the human soul did not possess an unlimited power of differentiation from the Infinite, then the Infinite would not be reflected in it, and consequently the Infinite Spirit would find no outlet for its *conscious* recognition of itself as the Life, Love, and Beauty which it is. We can never too deeply ponder the old esoteric definition of Spirit as "the Power which knows itself" : the secret of all things, past, present, and future is contained in these few words. The self-recognition or self-contemplation of Spirit is the primary movement out of which all creation proceeds, and the attainment in the individual of a fresh centre for self-recognition is what the Spirit *gains* in the process—this *gain* accruing to the Spirit is what is referred to in the parables where the lord is represented as receiving increase from his servants.

When the individual perceives this relation between himself and Infinite Spirit, he finds that he has been raised from a position of slavery to one of reciprocity. The Spirit cannot do without him any more than he can do without the Spirit : the two are as necessary to each other as the two poles of an electric battery. The Spirit is the unlimited essence of Love, Wisdom, and Power, all three in one undifferentiated and waiting to be differentiated by *appropriation*, that is, by the individual *claiming* to be the channel of their differentiation. It only requires the claim to be made with the recognition that by the Law of Being it is bound to be answered, and the right feeling, the right seeing, and the right working for the particular matter we have in hand will flow in quite naturally. Our old enemies, doubt and fear, may seek to bring us back under bondage to Baali, but our new stand-point for the recognition of the All-originating Spirit as being absolutely unified with ourselves must always

be kept resolutely in mind; for, short of this, we
are not working on the creative level—we are
creating, indeed, for we can never divest ourselves
of our creative power, but we are creating in the
image of the old limiting and destructive conditions, and this is merely perpetuating the cosmic
Law of Averages, which is just what the individual
has to rise superior to. The creative level is
where new laws begin to manifest themselves in a
new order of conditions, something transcending
our past experiences and thus bringing about a
real advance; for it is no advance only to go on in
the same old round even if we kept at it for cen-
turies: it is the steady go-ahead nature of the
Spirit that has made the world of to-day an improvement upon the world of the pterodactyl and
the icthiosaurus, and we must look for the same
forward movement of the Spirit from its new starting-point in ourselves.

Now it is this special, personal, and individual
relation of the Spirit to ourselves which is typified
by the names Ishi and Hephzibah. From this
stand-point we may say that as the individual wakes
up to the oneness with the Spirit, the Spirit wakes
up to the same thing. It becomes conscious of
itself through the consciousness of the individual,
and thus is solved the paradox of individual self-
recognition by the Universal Spirit, without which

no *new*-creative power could be exercised and all
things would continue to proceed in the old merely
cosmic order. It is of course true that in the
merely generic order the Spirit must be present in
every form of Life, as the Master pointed out when
He said that not a sparrow falls to the ground
without " the Father." But as the sparrows He alluded to had been shot and were on sale at a price
which shows that this was the fate of a good many
of them, we see here precisely that stage of manifestation where the Spirit has not woke up to individual self-recognition, and remains at the lower
level of self-recognition, that of the generic or race-
spirit. The Master's comment, " Ye are of more
value than many sparrows " points out this difference : in us the generic creation has reached the
level which affords the conditions for the waking up
of the Spirit to self-recognition in the Individual.

And we must bear in mind that all this is perfectly natural. There is no posing or straining after
effect about it. If *you* have to pump up the Life,
who is going to put the Life into you to pump it?
Therefore it is spontaneous or nothing. That is
why the Bible speaks of it as the free gift of God.
It cannot be anything else. You cannot originate
the originating force; it must originate you : but
what you can do is to distribute it. Therefore immediately you experience any sense of friction be

sure there is something wrong somewhere; and since God can never change, you may be sure that the friction is being caused by some error in your own thinking—you are limiting the Spirit in some way : set to work to find out what it is. It is always *limiting* the Spirit that does this. You are tying it down to conditions somewhere, saying it is bound by reason of some existing forms. The remedy is to go back to the original starting point of the Cosmic Creation and ask, Where were the pre-existing forms that dictated to the Spirit then? Then because the Spirit never changes it is *still the same,* and is just as independent of existing conditions now as it was in the beginning; and so we must pass over all existing conditions, however apparently adverse, and go straight to the Spirit as the originator of new forms and new conditions. This is real New Thought, for it does not trouble about the old things, but is going straight ahead from where we are now. When we do this, just trusting the Spirit, and not laying down the particular details of its action—just telling it what we want without dictating *how* we are to get it—we shall find that things will open out more and more clearly day by day both on the inner and the outer plane. Remember that the Spirit is alive and working here and now, for if ever the Spirit is to get from the past into the future it must be by passing through the present; therefore what you have to do is to acquire the habit of living direct from the Spirit here and now. You will soon find that this is a matter of personal intercourse, perfectly natural and not requiring any abnormal conditions for its production. You just treat the Spirit as you would any other kind-hearted sensible person, remembering that it is always there—" closer than hands and feet," as Tennyson says—and you will gradually begin to appreciate its reciprocity as a very practical fact indeed.

This is the relation of Hephzibah to Ishi, and is that worship in Spirit and in truth which needs neither the temple in Jerusalem nor yet in Samaria for its acceptance, for the whole world is the temple of the Spirit and you yourself its sanctuary. Bear this in mind, and remember that nothing is too great or too small, too interior or too external, for the Spirit's recognition and operation, for the Spirit is itself both the Life and the Substance of all things and it is also Self-recognition from the stand-point of your own individuality; and therefore, because the Self-recognition of Spirit is the Life of the creative process, you will, by simply trusting the Spirit to work according to its own nature, pass more and more completely into that New Order which proceeds from the thought of Him who says, " Behold I make all things new."

THE SHEPHERD AND THE STONE.

THE metaphor of the Shepherd and the Sheep is of constant occurrence throughout the Bible and naturally suggests the idea of the guiding, guarding, and feeding both of the individual sheep and of the whole flock and it is not difficult to see the spiritual correspondence of these things in a general sort of way. But we find that the Bible combines the metaphor of the Shepherd with another metaphor that of " the Stone," and at first sight the two seem rather incongruous.

" From thence is the Shepherd the Stone of Israel," says the Old Testament (Genesis xlix. 24), and Jesus calls himself both " The Good Shepherd " and " The Stone which the builders rejected." The Shepherd and the Stone are thus identified and we must therefore seek the interpretation in some conception which combines the two. A shepherd suggests Personal care for the welfare of the sheep, and an intelligence greater than theirs. A stone suggests the idea of Building, and consequently of measurement, adaptation of parts to whole, and progressive construction according to plan. Combining these two conceptions we get the idea of the building of an edifice whose stones are persons, each taking their more or less conscious part in the construction—thus a building, not constructed from without, but self-forming by a principle of growth from within under the guidance of a Supreme Wisdom permeating the whole and conducting it stage by stage to ultimate completeness.   This points to a Divine Order in human affairs with which we may more or less consciously co-operate: both to our personal advantage and also to the further- ance of the great scheme of human evolution as a whole; the ultimate purpose being to establish in *all* men that principle of "The Octave" to which I have already alluded; and in proportion as some adumbration of this principle is realized by individu- als and by groups of individuals they specialize the law of race-development, even though they may not be aware of the fact, and so come under a *spe- cialized* working of the fundamental Law, which thus differentiates them from other individuals and nationalities, as by a peculiar guidance, producing higher developments which the merely generic op- eration of the Law could not.

Now if we keep steadily in mind that, though the purpose, or Law of Tendency, or the Originating Spirit must always be universal in its nature, it must necessarily be individual in its operation, we shall see that this universal purpose can only be accomplished through the instrumentality of specific means. This results from the fundamental proposition that the Universal can only work on the plane of the Particular by becoming the individual and particular; and when we grasp the conception that the merely generic operation of the Creative Law has now brought the human race as far as it can, that is to say it has completely evolved the merely natural *genus homo*, it follows that if any further development is to take place it can only be by the co-operation of the individual himself. Now it is the spread of this individual co-operation that the forward movement of the Spirit is leading us to, and it is the gradual extension of this universal principle that is alluded to in the prophecy of Daniel regarding the Stone cut out without hands that spreads until it fills the whole earth (Daniel ii. 34 and 44). According to the interpretation given by Daniel, this Stone is the emblem of a spiritual Kingdom, and the identity of the Stone and the Shepherd indicates that the Kingdom of the Stone must be also the Kingdom of the Shepherd; and the Master, who identified himself with both the Stone and the Shepherd, emphatically declared that this Kingdom was, in its essence, an interior Kingdom—"the Kingdom of Heaven is within you." We must look for its foundation therefore, in a spiritual principle or mental law inherent in the constitution of all men but waiting to be brought into fuller development by more accurate compliance with its essential requirements; which is precisely the method by which science has evoked powers from the laws of nature which were undreamt of in former ages; and in like manner the recognition of our true relation to the Universal Spirit, which is the source of all individual being, must lead to an advance both for the race and for the individual such as we can at present scarcely form the faintest idea of, but which we dimly apprehend through the intuition and speak of as the New Order. The approach of this New Order is everywhere making itself vaguely felt; it is, as the French say, in the air, and the very vagueness and mystery attending it is causing a feeling of unrest as to what form it may assume. But to the student of Spiritual Law this should not be the case. He knows that the Form is always the expression of the Spirit, and therefore, since he is in touch with the forward movement of the Spirit, he knows that he himself will always be harmoniously included in any form of development which the Great Forward Movement may take. This is the practical and personal benefit arising from the realization of the Principle which is symbolized under the two-fold metaphor of the Shepherd and the Stone. and in all those new developments which are perhaps even now within measurable distance, we can rest on the knowledge that we are under the care of a kind Shepherd, and under the formation of a wise Master Builder.

But the principle of the Shepherd and the Stone is not something hitherto unheard of which is only to come into existence in the future. If there were no manifestations of this principle in the past, we might question whether there were any such principle at all; but a careful study of the subject will show us that it has been at work all through the ages, sometimes in modes more immediately bearing the aspect of the Shepherd, and sometimes in modes more immediately bearing the aspect of the Stone, though the one always implies the other, for they are the same thing seen from different points of view. The subject is one of immense interest, but covering such a wide range of study that all I can do here is to point out that such a field of investigation exists and is worth exploration; and the exploration brings its reward with it, not only by putting us in possession of the key to the history of the past, but by showing us that it is the key to the history of the future also, and furthermore by making evident on a large scale the working of the same principle of Spiritual Law by cooperation with which we may facilitate the process of our own individual evolution. It thus adds a

vivid interest to life, giving us something worth
looking forward to and introducing us to a personal
future which is not limited by the proverbial three-
score years and ten.

Now, we have seen that the first stage in the
Creative Process is always that of Feeling—a reach-
ing-out by the Spirit in a particular direction, and
therefore we may look for something of the same
kind in the development of the great principle
which we are now considering. And we find this
first vague movement of this great principle in the
intuitions of a particular race which appears from
time immemorial to have combined the two characteristics of nomad wandering with their flocks and
herds and the symbolization of their religious be-
liefs in monuments of stone. The monuments
themselves have taken different forms in different
countries and ages, but the identity of their symbolism becomes clear under careful investigation.
Together with this symbolism we always find the
nomad character of the builders and that they are
invested with an aura of mystery and romance such
as we find nowhere else, though we always find it
surrounding these builders, even in countries so far
apart as India and Ireland. Then, as we pass beyond the merely monumental stage, we find threads
of historical evidence connecting the different
branches of this race, increasing in their complexity

and strengthening in their cumulative force as we go on, until at last we are brought to the history of the age in which we live; and finally most remarkable affinities of language put the finishing touch to the mass of proofs which can be gathered along all these different lines. In this magic circle countries so remote from one another as Ireland and Greece, Egypt and India, Palestine and Persia, are brought into close contiguity—a similar tradition, and even a similar nomenclature, unite the mysterious builders of the Great Pyramid with the equally mysterious builders of the Round Towers of Ireland—and the Great Pyramid itself, perhaps antedating the call of Abraham, re-appears as the official seal of the United States; while tradition traces the crowning-stone in Westminster Abbey back to the time of Solomon's temple and even earlier. For the most part the erewhile wanderers are now settled in their destined homes, but the Anglo-Saxon race—the People of the Corner-Stone—are still the pioneers among the nations, and there is something esoteric in the old joke that when the North Pole is reached a Scotchman will be found there. And not least in the chain of evidence is the link afforded by a tribe who are wanderers still, the Gipsies with their duplicate of the Pyramid in the pack of cards—a volume which has been called " The Devil's Picture Book " by those who know it only in its misuse and inversion, but which when interpreted in the light of the knowledge we are now gaining, affords a signal instance of that divine policy by which as St. Paul says, God employs the foolish things of this world to confute the wise; while a truer apprehension of the Gipsies themselves indicates their unmistakable connection with that race who through all its wanderings has ever been the guardian of the Stone.

In these few paragraphs I have only been able to point out very briefly the broad lines of enquiry into a subject of national importance to the British and American peoples, and which interests us personally, not only as members of these nations, but as affording proof on the largest scale of the same specialization of universal laws which each of us has to effect individually for ourself. But whether the process be individual or national it is always the same, and is the translation to the very highest plane—that of the All-originating Life itself—of the old maxim that " Nature will obey us exactly in proportion as we first obey Nature "; it is the old parable of the lord who, finding his servants girt and awaiting him, then girds himself and serves them (Luke xii. 35 to 37). The nation or the individual who thus realizes the true principle of the Shepherd and the Stone, comes under a special Divine guidance and protection, not by a favouritism incompatible with the conception of universal Law, but by the very operation of the Law itself. They have come into touch with its higher possibilities, and to recur to an analogy which I have already employed, they learn to make their iron float by the very same law by which it sinks; and so they become the flock of the Great Shepherd and the building of the Great Architect, and each one, however insignificant his or her sphere may appear, becomes a sharer in the great work, and by a logical consequence begins to grow on new lines of development for the simple reason that a new principle necessarily produces new modes of manifestation. If the reader will think over these things he will see that the promises contained in the Bible, whether national or personal, are nothing else than statements of the universal law of Cause and Effect applied to the inmost principles of our being, and that therefore it is not mere rhapsody, but the figurative expression of a great truth when the Psalmist says "The Lord is my Shepherd," and "Thou art my God and the Rock of my salvation."

SALVATION IS OF THE JEWS.

WHAT does this saying of the Master's mean? Certainly not a mere arrogant assumption in favour of His own nationality—such an idea is negatived, not only by the universality of all His other teaching, but also by the very instruction in which these words occur, for He declared that the Jewish temple was equally with the Samaritan of no account in the matter. He said that the true worship was purely spiritual and entirely independent of places and ceremonies, while at the same time He emphasized the Jewish expectation of a Messiah, so that in this teaching we are met by the paradox of a universal principle combined with what at first sight appears like a tribal tradition quite incompatible with any recognition of the universal reign of law. How to reconcile these apparent opposites, therefore, seems to be the problem which He here sets before us. Its solution is to be found in that principle which I have endeavoured to elucidate throughout these lectures, the specializing of universal law. Opinions may differ as to whether the Bible narrative of the birth of Christ is to be taken

literally or symbolically, but as to the spiritual principle involved there can, I think, be no difference
of opinion. It is that of the specialization by the
individual of the generic relation of the soul to the
Infinite Spirit from which it proceeds. The relation itself is universal and results from the very
nature of the creative process, but the law of the
universal relation admits of particular specialization
exactly in the same way as all other natural laws—
it is simpy applying to the supreme Law of Life the
same method by which we have learnt to make iron
float, that is to say by a fuller recognition of what
the Law is in itself. Whatever other meanings we
may apply to the name Messiah, it undoubtedly
stands for the absolutely perfect manifestation in
the individual of all the infinite possibilities of the
Principle of Life.

Now it was because this grand ideal is the basis
on which the Hebrew nationality was founded that
Jesus made this statement. This foundation had
been lamentably misconceived by the Jewish people;
but nevertheless, however imperfectly, they still
held by it, and from them this ideal has spread
throughout the Christian world. Here also it continues to be lamentably misconceived, nevertheless
it is still retained, and only needs to be recognized
in its true light as a universal principle, instead of
an unintelligible dogma, to become the salvation of

the world. Hence, as affording the medium through which this supreme ideal has been preserved and spread, it is true that "Salvation is of the Jews."

Their fundamental idea was right but their apprehension of it was wrong—that is why the Master at the same time sweeps away the national worship of the temple and preserves the national idea of the Messiah; and this is equally true of the Christian world at the present day. If salvation is anything real it must have its cause in some law, and if there is a law it must be founded upon some universal principle: therefore it is this principle which we must seek if we would understand this teaching of the Master's.

Now whether we take the Bible story of the birth of Christ literally or symbolically, it teaches one great lesson. It teaches that the All-originating Spirit is the true Parent of the individual both in soul and body. This is nothing else than realizing from the stand-point of the individual what we cannot help realizing in regard to the original creation of the cosmos—it is the realization that the All-originating Spirit is at once the Life and the Substance in each individual here and now, just as it must have been in the origin of all things. Human parentage counts for nothing—it is only the channel through which Universal Spirit has acted for the concentration of an individual centre; but the ultimate cause of that centre, both in life and substance, continues at every moment to be the One same Originating Spirit.

This recognition cuts away the root of all the power of the negative, and so in principle it delivers us from all evil, for the root of evil is the denial of the power of the Spirit to produce good. When we realize that the Spirit is finding its own individualization in us in its two-fold essence as Life and Substance, then we see that it must be both able and willing to create for us all good. The only limit is that which we ourselves impose by denying its operation, and when we realize the inherent creativeness of Spirit we find that there is no reason why we should stop short at any point and say that it can go no further. Our error is in looking on the life of the body as separate from the life of the Spirit, and this error is met by the consideration that, in its ultimate nature, Substance must emanate from Spirit and is nothing else than the record of Spirit's conception of itself as finding expression in space and time. And when this becomes clear it follows that Substance need not be taken into calculation at all. The material form stands in the same relation to Spirit that the image projected on the screen stands to the slide in the lantern. If we wish to change the exhibited subject we do not manipulate the reflection on the screen, but we alter the slide; and in like manner, when we come to realize the true nature of the creative process, we learn that the exterior things are to be changed by a change of the interior spiritual attitude. Our spiritual attitude will always be determined by our conception of our relation to God or Infinite Spirit; and so when we begin to see that this relation is one of absolute reciprocity—that it is the self-recognition of Infinite Spirit from our own centre of consciousness—then we find that the whole Secret of Life consists in simple reliance upon the All-creating Spirit as consciously identifying itself with us. It has, so to say, awakened to a new mode of self-recognition peculiar to ourselves, in which we individually form the centre of its creative energy. To realize this is to specialize the Principle of Life. The logic of it is simple. We have found that the originating movement of Spirit from which all creation proceeds can only be Self-contemplation. Then, since the Original Spirit cannot change its nature its self-contemplation through our own minds must be as creative in, for, and through us as it ever was in the beginning; and consequently we find the original creative process repeated in ourselves and directed by the conscious thought of our own minds.

In all this there is no place for the consideration

of outward conditions, whether of body or circumstances; for they are only effects and not the cause;
and therefore when we reach this stand-point we
cease to take them into our calculations. Instead
we employ the method of self-contemplation,
knowing that this is the creative method, and so we
contemplate ourselves as allied to the infinite Love
and Wisdom of the Divine Spirit which will take
form through our conscious thought, and so act
creatively as a Special Providence entirely devoted
to guarding, guiding, providing for, and illuminating us. The whole thing is perfectly natural when
seen from a clear recognition of what the creative
working of Spirit must be in itself; and when it is
realized in this perfectly natural manner all strain
and effort to compel its action ceases—we are at
one with the All-creating Power which has now
found a new centre in ourselves from which to
continue its creative work to more perfect manifestation than could be attained through the unspe-
cialized generic conditions of the merely cosmic
order.

Now this is what Messiah stands for, and therefore it is written that " to them gave He power to
become sons of God, even to as many as believe on
His Name." This " belief " is the recognition of a
universal principle and personal reliance upon it as
a law which cannot be broken; for it is the Law of

the whole creative process specialized in our own individuality. Then, too, however great may be the mystery, the removal and cleansing away of all sin follows as an essential part of this realization of new life; and it is in this sense that we may read all that the Bible tells us on this aspect of the subject. The *principle* of it is Love; for when we are reunited to the Parent Spirit in mutual confidence and love, what room is there on either side for any remembrance of our past failures?

This, then, is what Messiah stands for to the individual; but if we can conceive a nation based upon such a recognition of its special relation to the Directing Power of the Universe, such a people must of necessity become the leader of the nations, and those who oppose it must fail by a self-destructive principle inherent in the very nature of the position they take up. The leadership resulting from such a national self-recognition, will not be based upon conquest and compulsion, but will come naturally. Other nations will enquire the reason for the phenomenal success and prosperity of the favoured people, and finding this reason in a universal Law, they will begin to apply the same law in the same manner, and thus the same results will spread from country to country until at last the whole earth will be full of the glory of the Lord. And such a nation, and rather company of nations, exists. To trace its present development from its ancient beginnings is far beyond the scope of this volume, and still more to speculate upon its further growth; but to my readers on both sides of the Atlantic I may say that this people is the Anglo-Saxon race throughout the world. I write these lines upon the historic Hill of Tara; this will convey a hint to many of my readers. At some future time I may enlarge upon this subject; but at present my aim is merely to suggest some lines of thought arising from the Master's saying that " Salvation is of the Jews."